Women with Serious Mental Illness

Women with Serious Mental Illness

Gender-Sensitive and
Recovery-Oriented Care

LAUREN MIZOCK AND ERIKA CARR

OXFORD
UNIVERSITY PRESS

OXFORD
UNIVERSITY PRESS

Oxford University Press is a department of the University of Oxford. It furthers
the University's objective of excellence in research, scholarship, and education
by publishing worldwide. Oxford is a registered trade mark of Oxford University
Press in the UK and certain other countries.

Published in the United States of America by Oxford University Press
198 Madison Avenue, New York, NY 10016, United States of America.

Library of Congress Cataloging-in-Publication Data
Names: Mizock, Lauren, author. | Carr, Erika, author.
Title: Women with serious mental illness : gender-sensitive and
recovery-oriented care / Lauren Mizock, & Erika Carr.
Description: New York : Oxford University Press, 2021. |
Includes bibliographical references and index.
Identifiers: LCCN 2020022726 (print) | LCCN 2020022727 (ebook) |
ISBN 9780190922351 (paperback) | ISBN 9780190922375 (epub) |
ISBN 9780190922382
Subjects: LCSH: Women with mental disabilities. | Women with mental
disabilities—Social conditions. | Women with mental
disabilities—Counseling of.
Classification: LCC HV3009.5.W65 M59 2021 (print) |
LCC HV3009.5.W65 (ebook) | DDC 362.2082—dc23
LC record available at https://lccn.loc.gov/2020022726
LC ebook record available at https://lccn.loc.gov/2020022727

9 8 7 6 5 4 3 2 1

Printed by Marquis, Canada

CONTENTS

Acknowledgments vii

1. Introduction 1

2. History of the Mistreatment of Women with Serious Mental Illness 6

3. Women with Serious Mental Illness, Resilience, and the
   Recovery Movement 24

4. Motherhood, Family, and Relationships for Women with Serious
   Mental Illness 45

5. Work and Class Among Women with Serious Mental Illness 70

6. Cultural Factors Among Women with Serious Mental Illness: Race, Gender,
   Sexuality, and Spirituality 91

7. Trauma and Sexual Objectification of Women with Serious Mental Illness 113

8. Preventing Retraumatization of Women with Serious Mental Illness 131

9. Women's Empowerment and Recovery-Oriented Care: A New
   Intervention Model 149

About the Authors 161
Bibliography 163
Index 189

ACKNOWLEDGMENTS

The contents of this book were developed with the support of Fielding Graduate University. The authors are also grateful for the support of the Center for Psychiatric Rehabilitation at Boston University, Fielding Graduate University, and Yale Medical School, as well as graduate students at Fielding Graduate University for assistance with adjacent research to this project. Finally, we thank our husbands, parents, in-laws, childcare providers, and children for their support and patience with our "book baby."

Introduction

Many mental health providers are unaware that they commonly serve women with serious mental illness (SMI). These clients include the woman with severe depression who cannot get out of bed in the morning; or the woman with complex post-traumatic stress disorder (PTSD) who misses work because of paralyzing flashbacks. She is the woman with schizophrenia who avoids bathing because she fears she is being watched; or the woman with bipolar disorder whose episodes of unpredictable behavior have estranged her from her family.

SMI specifically refers to a major mental health problem leading to significant impairment in areas of work, school, social functioning, and/or activities of daily living. While many practitioners have worked with women with SMI, they are often not thinking about their clients through this lens. The unique clinical considerations and experiences of these women are often overlooked in clinical settings, research, and training. Moreover, the impact of their intersecting identities (i.e., racial-ethnic, sexual, socioeconomic, religious) on their mental health is rarely explored in research, training, or practice.

There is a need for more research on therapy for women with SMI, and much of the current literature could benefit from an update. Little has been written in this area for some time. In 1997, Maxine Harris and Christine Landis edited the volume *Sexual Abuse in the Lives of Women Diagnosed with Serious Mental Illness*. This book provided a much-needed focus on the experience of sexual exploitation and mistreatment among this population. Prior to her death in 2005, Carol Mowbray also researched the needs of women with SMI in many of her articles on mental health services for mothers, young adult women, and female caregivers. Much of the recent literature on women with SMI focuses on mothers (National Research Council and Institute of Medicine, 2009; Reupert, Maybery, Nicholson, Gopfert, & Seeman, 2015), including a newer book entitled *Motherhood, Mental Illness and Recovery* (2013). Moreover, much of the extant research focuses on women with a specific diagnosis or less severe notions of mental illness such as mild to moderate anxiety and depressive disorders. More research is needed that concentrates on the broader concerns and experiences of one of the primary populations being served in mental health settings.

Given our passion for providing psychotherapy to women with SMI, this gap in the literature has called us to action. We realized our shared commitment to the specific interests, needs, and experiences of women who experience SMI in our work for the American Psychological Association (APA). We saw that the stories of the inspiring women we served were missing from publications and training programs, and decided that this topic could benefit from a feminist psychology perspective. And so, we set forth to develop a task force within the Society for the Psychology of Women (Division 35) of the APA to raise awareness of this group. We began a professional collaboration to develop this book to fill this gap in the literature and offer a new resource to providers, researchers, trainees, and others. With this book, we hope to breathe new life into an important topic from a gender-sensitive and recovery-oriented perspective.

This framework of this book will include feminist theory, the concept of intersectionality of oppression, and the model of recovery-oriented care. We will emphasize the multiple social identities and experiences of women with SMI that contribute to complex experiences of stigma, access to care, and recovery. We will explore the elevated rates of abuse, trauma, poverty, and homelessness encountered by these women. Women with SMI have been desexualized, retraumatized, and hypersexualized in mental health settings, or objectified by their diagnoses instead of being validated for their valued roles and strengths as mothers, partners, and members of a family or community.

Language is particularly salient in this book. "SMI" may not be the terminology that feminist therapists find familiar, comfortable, or preferred. As multicultural feminist therapists, we have often moved away from words that further pathologize already stigmatized identities. We have discussed this terminology dilemma with many colleagues who also specialize in therapy for women with SMI. What we have found is that some of our clients favor the term "SMI," finding it a validating and accurate representation of their experience.

Alternative terms to SMI that are currently used in the field include "psychiatric disability" or "person in recovery." The former shares a focus on functioning with SMI. However, some of our therapy clients and research participants have described this term as limiting by labeling their identities as disabled. The latter phrase, "person in recovery," has grown out of the ex-patients' movement of the 1970s, leading to the current recovery movement. In this context, recovery refers to the notion that people can live meaningful and satisfying lives in the face of SMI. The recovery movement shares many feminist values with principles that are anti-stigma, social justice-focused, strengths-based, and hope-centered. However, other practitioners and researchers might not be aware of this connotation of recovery, and may associate it with sobriety or symptom elimination. Furthermore, one may use the term "recovery" to refer to an approach toward coping with a mental health problem, as opposed to a name for one's condition. The connotation of the term "recovery" in this book is synergistic with the recovery-oriented care movement and mental health recovery. The recovery model puts forth that people with SMI have the right to pursue their dreams and live a life of meaning as they so define, beyond the effects of mental illness.

While the term "SMI" raises linguistic challenges, we use it in this book to call attention to the specific needs and experiences these women may have. Providing therapy to someone with mild depression, anxiety, or an "adjustment disorder" might look very different than providing therapy to someone who has difficulty functioning due to daily battles with belittling voices. In a previous work of one of our authors, this challenge of language and diagnosis is termed *diagnostic dialectic tension* (Mizock & Kaschak, 2015). The term captures that on the one hand, it is vital that therapists are empowering people with these experiences and avoid further stigma with regard to the use of mental health diagnoses. On the other hand, a diagnosis may be important to naming a mental health problem to foster awareness and professional communication and to identify appropriate care. Ultimately, each woman should be supported to choose a term for her mental health problem that feels appropriate and empowering to her. In this book, we will explain how therapists can work with women with SMI to identify their preferred language, which may change and evolve over time.

With our gender-sensitive focus in the book, we will bring attention to issues of sexism, misogyny, and power faced by women with SMI. Feminist therapy has come to be referred by some as *gender-sensitive therapy* in order to enhance inclusivity to other genders in this approach (Walker, 2009). Gender-sensitive therapy focuses on issues of empowerment, agency, and enhanced coping of the client in reaction to sources of oppression as they impact mental health. And gender oppression is a central factor that impacts the development and recovery from SMI among women.

For example, according to 2015 statistics from the National Institute of Mental Health, women are more likely to experience SMI than men (5% female; 3% male). Women experience higher rates of victimization and sexual trauma that impact their mental health (Jonikas, Laris, & Cook, 2003; Mowbray, Nicholson, & Bellamy, 2003). Women with SMI are more likely to face single parenthood and caretaking responsibilities (Jonikas et al., 2003; Mowbray et al., 2003). Though some statistics suggest that men with SMI tend to have higher rates of homelessness than their female counterparts, other estimates suggest that young women face greater rates of homelessness (36% female; 26% male) and women with children face particular housing barriers and risks of homelessness (Davis & Vander Stoep, 1997; Jonikas et al., 2003; Kidd et al., 2013). However, women with SMI experience unique strengths in contrast to their male counterparts, including a greater likelihood of being partnered and socially connected—important protective factors to mental health challenges (Kidd et al., 2013).

Our examination of gender issues will also include treatment issues. Women have also commonly encountered insensitivity, bias, and exploitation from the mental health professionals they have sought for help (Ussher, 2011). Diagnosticians appear to be commonly biased by stereotypes of women in mental health care, such as over-diagnosing affective and personality disorders and under-diagnosing substance abuse problems and PTSD (Eriksen & Kress, 2008;

Mueser et al., 1998; Seeman, 2000). Initial theories on gender differences in men and women with SMI were often attributed to biology, reinforcing gender bias (Gove, 1980). Women with SMI have historically been identified as "mad" when not conforming to societal norms or have been designated as having inherent, inferior status (Ussher, 2011).

We will address this history of mistreatment of women with SMI in the next chapter—both in the broader society, as well as in the mental health system in the United States and Western Europe. We will discuss the ways in which labeling women as "mad" has marginalized women, while those with actual psychiatric symptoms have been mistreated or overlooked in mental health care. We will also discuss trends in misdiagnosis, institutionalization, and exploitation of women who have sought mental health treatment throughout time.

We focus on the recovery movement in Chapter 3, and the impact of this model on the care of women with SMI. We will describe how the recovery perspective involves a holistic view of the person, with talents and strengths beyond the dehumanizing identity of "mental patient." We will also focus on the effect of stigma in the lives of people with SMI and how this experience adds suffering to the experience of SMI. We will review the various components of recovery, including the renewal of hope and the importance of pursuing valued social roles.

In Chapter 4, we explore issues of relationships, family, and motherhood for women with SMI. Given the traditional expectations of women to be mothers and partners, we will explore how the effects of SMI can interfere with these roles and can impact one's sense of womanhood and personhood. We will address how motherhood is a valued and normalizing social role and can serve as a facilitator to recovery. We will explore how motherhood and other relationships can serve as a context for recovery.

We will present the literature on experiences of work, class, and poverty among women with SMI in Chapter 5. We will examine financial barriers these women face and the associated effects on their recovery journey. We will propose clinical strategies for handling these challenges in mental health care and supporting the financial wellness and employment interests of women with SMI.

In Chapter 6 we will explore a number of cultural issues in the lives of women with SMI. We will include the experiences of women of color with SMI who encounter racism, misogyny, homophobia, and mental illness stigma. We will also examine issues of religion and spirituality that might offer a source of strength and empowerment.

We will apply sexual objectification theory to the sexual exploitation of women who experience SMI in Chapter 7. We will describe the ways in which culture sexually objectifies the bodies of these women. Both acute and insidious examples of these experiences will be explored, as well as the high incidence of sexual abuse, assault, and exploitation that heighten the likelihood of PTSD among these women. Here we will also present the clinical applications for working with women who have had sexually objectifying experiences.

In Chapter 8 we will discuss the complex concerns that occur when women with SMI encounter retraumatization in treatment settings. The chapter will provide an overview of these challenges, various strengths within treatment settings, and strategies for incorporating trauma-informed care and psychological safety within psychiatric settings.

In the final chapter, we will introduce the *Women's Empowerment and Recovery-Oriented Care* (WE-ROC) model, a culturally competent framework that includes feminist and recovery frameworks in order to best engage with women with SMI and their unique needs and experiences. We will also mention the potential applications of this gender-sensitive intervention for men with SMI who face challenges associated with traditional masculinity, including barriers to help-seeking and health-promoting behaviors.

To make the book most useful to our readers, we include clinical strategies lists, worksheets, discussion questions, activities, tables, diagrams, case vignettes, and a resource appendix throughout the chapters. These additions make the book a valuable tool for clinical work, research, and training. Graduate students, trainers, practitioners, and other helpers can complete discussion questions, activities, and worksheets on their own, in classes, in training seminars, or when working with clients.

With this book we envision new directions for the care of women with SMI by attending to the complex, multiple identities and needs of women with SMI. We believe this perspective can help to understand the effects of marginalization and privilege on women's mental health. We hope to work toward prevention of the mistreatment of women with SMI and to provide therapy that is sensitive to identity and power. We should note that this book focuses on psychosocial aspects of the recovery process and psychological care. While the medical and public health perspectives are also important, we will primarily address this topic through our professional lens as clinical psychologists. For further information on medical, biological, and pharmacologic aspects of care with this population as well as public health models, we direct our readers to other excellent resources (see Casper, 2008; Levin & Becker, 2010; Lewis-Hall, Williams, Panetta, & Herrera, 2002).

As feminist psychologists, we see the needs of women with SMI as a social justice issue. We believe that all individuals have the right to safety, adequate resources, self-determination, and equity. We have been moved by our clinical experiences with these women to speak out about the injustices they experience and associated effects on their recovery. We hope this book inspires conversations and activism that can enhance psychology and medical training and inspire policy that supports the rights of women with SMI. We encourage you to use this book to traverse the traditional models of psychotherapy and effect social change in your own personal and professional community.

2

History of the Mistreatment of Women with Serious Mental Illness

In researching the history of the treatment of women with serious mental illness (SMI), there was plenty of evidence to support the central thesis of this book: Women with SMI face a double jeopardy to their welfare as a result of sexism and psychiatric stigma. However, a surprising discovery emerged. It was difficult to find out how women with SMI were treated at all because so many women were deemed mentally ill. Rather than having a mental illness, many of these women were assigned this label because they defied social roles, or functioned as scapegoats for the problems of their communities. Ironically, many women who appeared to have genuine psychiatric symptoms were often overlooked in mental health care. Whether all women who were considered mentally ill truly had this condition may be impossible to divine at this point in time. Nevertheless, much can be learned from how gender norms shaped the mental health treatment of women in the past.

This chapter will include relevant mental health trends in the treatment of women in the Western world for the last several centuries. This chronicle will span from such exotic tragedies as the mass hysteria of witch hunts, to gynecological surgeries thought to cure insanity. Luckily there have been critics of misogynistic treatments throughout these times, and their struggles for justice will be highlighted in this account. We will also see how themes in the mistreatment of women's mental health endure into the present day.

THEORIES ON THE HISTORY OF WOMEN'S MADNESS

A chapter on the history of women's mental health treatment would not be complete without a nod to the feminist critics who tackled this history before and developed key perspectives on this topic. Psychologist Phyllis Chesler contributed what has been called the *Cheslerian thesis* (Tomes, 1990) in her book *Women's Madness* (1991). Another psychologist, Jane Ussher, also wrote a seminal work in this area, *Women's Madness: Misogyny or Mental Illness?* (1991). Chesler and Ussher presented radical arguments on the diagnosing of women with mental illness throughout history. They redefined women's "symptoms" as stress reactions to their oppression or signs of protest against it. Chesler and Ussher theorized that women's treatments for madness were attempts to subdue their uprising. To this effect, Ussher (1991) wrote:

> . . . what we call 'madness' is the product of systematic and regulated discursive practice, whose genealogy can be historically traced to show their connections with other discourses, such as that of 'witch' or 'hysteric'. We can prise apart the meanings and assumptions fused together in the ways we understand women's madness in order to see our present practices as historically determined phenomena rather than as timeless and incontrovertible facts. Such an analysis of the construction of the modern form of women's madness is a prerequisite for understanding and bringing about change. (p. 288)

The historian Nancy Tomes (1990) presented a different argument in a comprehensive chapter on this topic. Tomes maintained that many of the efforts of early psychiatry were relatively innocent and well-intentioned attempts to rectify women's mental health symptoms based on the medical thinking of that time, often at the request of female patients or their family members. Tomes argued that physicians sympathized with the stress of working-class mothers, understanding their mental illness as originating from too many offspring and exhaustion from excessive domestic labor. However, Tomes also contended that the problems of women's mental health treatment should not be forgotten:

> Recent historical work has begun to reconsider certain assumptions about the gender-madness nexus, and to reject oversimplified notions of women's liability to mental illness and victimization at the hands of male physicians. This new approach has resulted in a much more complex reading of women's experience as mental patients. But in rewriting the history of women and madness, historians must be careful not to overromanticize their subjects. While the madwoman may not have been a helpless victim of male hostility, she nonetheless suffered the burden not only of madness but of gender, a fact that we cannot afford to forget. (p. 171)

Elaine Showalter (1995), a feminist literary critic, wrote another important book in this area, *The Female Malady: Women, Madness, and English Culture, 1830–1980*. She painted a picture of history somewhere between the radical Cheslerian thesis and Tomes's more sympathetic depiction of the medical profession. Showalter highlighted the indisputable misogyny of the treatment of the suffragettes who were institutionalized and force-fed during hunger strikes. She

also showcased the humane physicians who cared for women with mental illness in asylums, contrasted with other concurrent punitive treatments of women's
madness or sexual desire.

Women with SMI were not the only victims of mistreatment in the mental
health world historically. Ussher (1991) spoke to past problems in the treatment
of men:

> So men may be mad—but are likely to be positioned as bad. They are likely
> to manifest their discontent or deviancy as criminals. Whilst women are
> positioned within the psychiatric discourse, men are positioned with the
> criminal discourse. We are regulated differently. (p. 10)

Showalter (1995) also explored torturous treatments of men in this history, which will be included in this chapter. Incidences such as these show that
women were not the only victims of rigid gender role expectations and inhumane
psychiatric care.

While the history of men's mental health treatment is outside the scope of this
chapter, these authors remind us that women were not the only victims of gender
bias. At the same time, male privilege appeared to protect men from mistreatment
in many cases. In the following sections, we will see how women's lack of power
was particularly damaging for the women who were labeled mentally ill. And with
a review of these feminist theories, we will take care to manage the fallacy of "pres-
entism" as we continue with this chapter—the bias to interpret past events with
current values. At the same time, we will willingly engage in the subjective construction of feminist interpretations of past practices in women's mental health in
order to inform our present-day implementation of gender-sensitive care.

EARLY VIEWS ON WOMEN'S MENTAL HEALTH

Relics of ancient times suggest that mental illness was often understood to result
from demonological possession or supernatural sorcery (Porter, 2002). Women
were predisposed to mental illness due to a biological weakness and suggesti-
bility to spiritual forces (Tasca et al., 2012). Women's mental illness could also be
a signal of sin or problems with reproduction.

One word described the mental illness of women (and often men) for
centuries: hysteria. The first medical document in ancient Egypt depicted symptoms
of seizures, suffocation, and fear of death, perhaps resembling symptoms of what
we now consider to be panic attacks (Tasca et al., 2012). Hippocrates (460–370
BCE) is believed to have officially coined the term in the fifth century BCE, linking
women's mental health problems with a wandering womb.

Hippocrates featured in the development of ancient Greek medicine with
his contribution of the humorism model. Physical and mental illnesses derived
from an imbalance in fluids in the body, the four humors. Women were prone
to imbalances in cold and wet humors, and vulnerable to developing uterine

sickness. This could be healed by several mechanisms: sexual activity and reproduction, manual manipulation of the uterus, or application of pungent and per-
fumed substances.

In Rome from the first century BCE to the second century CE, hysteria continued to be a key diagnosis assigned to women (Tasca et al., 2012). The Greek
physician Galen (130–210 CE) added to Hippocrates's theories of symptoms with
anxiety and more catatonic dispositions. Galen believed these could be treated
through herbs, purging, marriage, and reduced sexual excitement. In contrast, the
Greek physician Soranus, in the first and second century CE, viewed hysteria as a
result of problems with reproduction. Soranus's treatment was massage, exercise,
warm soaks, or sexual abstinence.

Ancient attributions of mental illness to women's reproductive systems and
sexual behavior represent essentialist, biological perspectives of gender and
mental health. Hysteria even continues to be used as a diagnosis in some areas of
the world. We will illuminate how these perspectives persist into modern times,
albeit in new iterations.

EARLY MODERN EUROPE AND COLONIAL UNITED STATES

Fast-forwarding to medieval Europe, a demonological view of mental illness
returned. Religious piety was central to culture, along with concepts of melancholia and hysteria (Tasca et al., 2012). Some female healers are worthy of note
in this history. Trotula de Ruggiero, an 11th-century female doctor in Salerno,
allegedly attributed hysteria to a lack of sexual activity and fulfillment of desire.
She treated hysteria with a prescription of mint, musk oil, and sexual activity.
Hildegard of Binge, an 11th-century female doctor from Germany, revisited
the humorism model. She viewed hysteria and melancholia as caused by ex-
cess of the black bile humor, as well as original sin, occurring among both men
and women.

In the 1200s, St. Thomas Aquinas proposed that mental illness developed among
women due to inherent inferiority, demonic possession, and witchcraft (Tasca
et al., 2012). As a result, many women were targeted who were identified with
hysteria or melancholia. Other women who were scapegoated for the seizures and
deaths of nearby adults and children were also persecuted. These women faced exorcism, torture, imprisonment, and murder. The demonological views of mental
illness reinvigorated the supernatural beliefs in mental illness from ancient times.
Hence, the cause of mental illness became a lack of faith and the handiwork of
the devil.

During the Renaissance era, from the 14th through 17th centuries, ancient
Greek writings on medicine were revived, valuing free will and moral reason. As
a result, biological explanations of hysteria reemerged (Tasca et al., 2012). In the
1600s, Descartes linked behavior and the body, contributing a more scientific understanding of mental illness. Physical and psychological etiologies predominated

in understandings of women with mental illness in these times. The cause became not just a wandering uterus but also the brain and nervous system.

The pendulum swung back to spiritual explanatory models of mental illness in Western Europe in the 17th and 18th centuries. This belief system extended to the early U.S. colonies, where religious fervor predominated and mental illness might be attributed to sin, lack of religious piety, or the devil (Tomes, 1990). Some have suggested that the victims of alleged witchcraft were experiencing symptoms of epilepsy, diabetes, or dissociative identity disorder (Sneddon, 2016).

During the Salem witch trials in New England, witch hunts developed under Puritanical religious fervor (Ushher, 1991). In the late 14th to 17th century, somewhere between hundreds of thousands and millions of mostly women were persecuted under the auspices of witchcraft. Due to poor records, it is difficult to ascertain the precise number of women who were executed. We do know that the witch trials were so dramatic in scope that they may rank in size with the genocides of the Holocaust and the Spanish Inquisition.

During this period, mental illness was interpreted as the work of evil spirits, stemming from a lack of religious piety (Ussher, 1991). Treatment entailed exorcism and other punishments like public stripping, gang rape, and execution. Women continued to be blamed for the illnesses that developed among various community members and children. Some witches were identified among melancholic or "sexually depraved" women. Others were holistic healers and midwives who occasionally performed abortions. Since women were barred from traditional medical training, many with interests in these areas practiced lay medicine. Other women who were vulnerable to witchcraft accusations were property owners, lesbians, survivors of domestic violence, or "proven masturbators."

In a blending of demonological and medical models, some believed that witchcraft could be cured through clitoridectomy, the surgical excision of the clitoris (Chessler, 2005). Danish physician Johann Weyer (1515–1588) has been viewed as an advocate for people with SMI during this era, and was credited with protecting those accused of witchcraft as mentally ill. The 19th-century French neurologist Jean-Martin Charcot (1825–1893) later claimed that the accused had hysteria and neurosis, causing the erratic behavior that led to their targeting as witches.

Ussher (1991) deconstructed the well-intentioned theory that the women executed for witchcraft were mentally ill. She argued that it remains unclear who among these women had a mental illness, if at all. Reports of hallucinations of women on trial for witchcraft could have been stories produced under torture. It is impossible to determine if these were actual symptoms of psychosis, or simply forced falsehoods. We might add that these women could have also experienced brief psychotic episodes induced by the extreme trauma and stress of their persecution. Ultimately, Ussher argued that attributing mental illness to these women constitutes victim blaming, rather than holding the persecutors accountable for the killing of tens of thousands of women.

INDUSTRIALIZATION AND THE VICTORIAN ERA

In the 18th and 19th centuries, women's gender roles became more traditionally domestic as a result of the effects of industrialization on labor (Tomes, 1990). Men went to work in factories and women stayed at home. Women came to be seen as more fragile and anxious, leading some to adopt the sick role, which also served as an escape from dreary domestic life. Gender roles influenced the understanding and expression of mental illness in new ways. Men's mental illness was ascribed to problem habits (e.g., alcoholism, substance abuse, hypersexuality) and women's to family, social, and moral issues. Insanity itself involved a problem in performing designated gender roles.

The trope of the madwoman in the attic replaced that of the madman in this era (Showalter, 1995). This was evidenced by the greater hospitalization of women at this time, as well as the fixation in medicine on the mental illnesses of women (Showalter, 1995; Tomes, 1990). Asylum "respites" could include confinement and treatments more painful than healing (Smith-Rosenberg & Brumberg, 1973; Tomes, 1990). Madness became medicalized rather than spiritualized. Mental illness became biomedical in nature rather than a deficit in devoutness or a supernatural affliction. Among the key features of women's mental health treatment were the growth of asylum psychiatry, gynecological surgery, and a number of newer diagnoses.

Asylum Psychiatry

In the Victorian era, Parliament in the United Kingdom created a public asylum system that was class-based and largely populated by paupers and men, as the wealthy had the options of home care or private institutions (Showalter, 1995). This changed by the mid-1850s, when women predominated in public asylums as well as in the outpatient clinics. However, many of the women in asylums were not mentally ill but were physically disabled or had a chronic illness. During this era, mental illness was often seen as having not only physical but also moral causes. Physical causes included intemperance, masturbation, brain injury, fever, and epilepsy. Moral causes included domestic problems, jealousy, excitement, and loss of property.

Women in the asylums were put to work with chores and handicrafts (Showalter, 1995). "Laundry therapy" was a treatment created during this time that was believed to prevent violence (though many would guess it would be more likely to incite it!). Men in the asylums were assigned to tasks involving more physical labor. As a result, they spent more time outdoors during the day, with shorter workdays brought on by sunset. Women were expected to toil at domestic tasks into the later hours by candlelight. Tomes (1990) demarcated the class disparities in the division of labor: Working-class women were appointed to wash clothing and linens, while middle-class women were expected to read and make crafts.

Chesler (2005) depicted private madhouses as places where wealthy men could warehouse wives they no longer wished to be married to. One example was Elizabeth Packard, a U.S. woman who was forcibly and legally institutionalized in Illinois in 1860 by her clergyman husband in spite of having no mental health issues. In Bible class, she taught that people are born good, not evil. Because of this transgression of "free religious inquiry," Packard was institutionalized for several years. This injustice became a key motivator for asylum reform.

In an article on sex and gender in the history of psychiatry, Hirshbein (2010) argued that attributing mental illness to gender factors in biology was a form of essentialism. This model underestimated the impact of sociocultural factors on women's mental health, and overestimated the effects of hormones and reproduction. Psychiatrists and neurologists reified these gender differences by admitting more and more women to asylums and outpatient neurology clinics. The higher incidences of schizophrenia, tertiary syphilis, and paranoia among men were often ignored. With biological essentialism came the gendering of emotion. For example, women were seen as not rational enough to become voters, much less politicians or other roles that came with power.

Showalter (1995) described the movement of Darwinian psychiatry of this era. Darwinian psychiatry included eugenics principles that people with SMI were genetically unfit to carry on the human race. These psychiatrists believed women passed on mental illness to their daughters. They committed feminist suffragettes for political activities, going on hunger strikes, or refusing to marry. There was also a focus on female nervous disorders, such as hysteria, neurasthenia, and a slew of other conditions that we will touch on, as well as the implementation of biological procedures that attempted to "rectify" the minds of women.

Gynecological Surgery

One biological procedure used on women at this time was gynecological surgery. Irregular menstruation was treated with medicines, baths, or leeches on genitals and thighs used to stave off the effects of mental illness (Showalter, 1995). Ovariectomies were also used to treat mental health issues in women and to prevent further pregnancies, which were thought to predispose a woman to lactational and puerperal (postpartum) insanity. Clitoridectomies and labiotomies were conducted to discourage masturbation, considered both a sign and cause of mental illness.

For example, the following obstetrical surgical case report from 1887 by Irish physician William K. M'Mordie, MD, detailed a surgery he performed to remove a woman's ovaries:

> S.J. aged thirty-three, married thirteen years and the mother of six children, accompanied by her family surgeon, Dr. Give, of Magh, consulted me on August 23, 1886. She had previously been confined to an asylum for the insane for some time. She was a confirmed masturbator, and performed the

act quite regardless of the presence of other people—even in the presence of her husband and children. After each performance she suffered from a paroxysm of excitement, followed by despondency. She stated she was quite unable to give up the habit. I advised the removal of the ovaries, as giving, in my opinion, the only hope of a cure for the pernicious habit. I also held out a hope that the operation might result in a permanent benefit to her mental condition. In this opinion Dr. Given concurred. I fully explained the nature of the operation both to the woman and her husband . . .

After the operation she only once attempted to interfere with her person. On December 9th her husband wrote:—"Her mind is not much improved, but she never interferes with herself." The woman stated she had contracted the habit of masturbation long before her mind was affected . . .

Now it seems to me that since the verdict of the profession is largely in favor of the removal of the ovaries for many physical derangements dependent upon menstruation, the same remedy should, a fortiori, be tried for those mental derangements which plainly arise, or seem to arise, from the same source. The objections to such remedy when applied for mental diseases, are, in fact, less valid than when it is resorted to for physical lesions. For, in the first place, an insane woman is no more a member of the body politic than a criminal; secondly, her death is always a relief to her dearest friends; thirdly, even in case of her recovery from her mental disease, she is liable to transmit the taint of insanity to her children, and to her children's children, for many generations. The removal, therefore, of the ovaries in such a case would tend to restore a woman to home and to society, and it would at the same time effectually bar her from having an insane offspring. (Goodell, 1882, p. 575)

This account shows that masturbation was regarded as a moral issue and sign of mental illness that could be quite distressing for women. The physician justified the ovariectomy as a treatment for insanity even though her mental health had not improved following the surgery. The patient was seen as failing to participate in society and in her gender roles, acting as a drain on her community. To add to all this was the sterilization that ensued from ovarian removal, preventing genetic transmission of insanity. If the women died, the physician reasoned that their death would be a relief to their friends and family.

Tomes (1990) critiqued understandings of gynecological surgery as attempts to silence the sexual desire and behavior of "unruly" women. Rather, medicalized perceptions of mental illness led to essentialist understandings of differences in men's and women's mental illness. Medical intervention was driven largely by physicians' attempts to improve their professional standing and treat women with legitimate gynecological problems. Tomes argued that extreme proponents of gynecological surgery were viewed as controversial in the psychiatric community, and were sometimes expelled from it, as in the following example.

The English physician Isaac Baker Brown (1811–1873) is an extreme case of practitioners of clitoridectomy and labiotomy (Showalter, 1995). Brown performed these surgeries on a wide range of women, believing mental illness was signaled by women who masturbated or were particularly sexually inclined. Also within his purview were women who shirked the domestic role, including nuns, nurses, and those seeking divorce. Brown was eventually barred from the Obstetrical Society of London in 1867. Though some physicians agreed that masturbation was a symptom of women's mental illness, gynecological surgery was often considered to be an unnecessary and drastic treatment.

Puerperal and Lactational Insanity

As previously mentioned, there were several types of insanity diagnosed among women. Although various causes of insanity were proposed, such as problems with the reproductive organs, pregnancy, or blood poisoning and inflammation, "treatment" was attempted through removal of the uterus and other areas of the reproductive system (Showalter, 1995). Physicians began to focus on physical causes of mental health problems among women within the reproductive organs, or "reflex" insanity (Theriot, 1989). Puerperal insanity took place in the six weeks after childbirth, while lactational insanity occurred several months after childbirth (Loudon, 1988). These diagnoses captured various states of melancholia, mania, and/or psychosis and attributed the symptoms to women's reproductive cycles.

At times, these insanities may have actually been delirium brought on by toxic infections and fever. At other times, they were simply "wastebasket" diagnoses assigned to women who displayed angry outbursts, lack of interest in their families, or shouting and aggressive behavior, all of which clashed with gender expectations (Showalter, 1995). Some diagnoses may have reflected what we now understand to be postpartum or peripartum psychosis and depression (Loudon, 1988). However, they were clearly over-diagnosed when compared to current prevalence rates.

In the latter part of the 19th century, physicians attributed puerperal insanity to the weakening of womanhood with societal change (Loudon, 1988). The modern woman was seen as too feeble to withstand labor unaided and was likely to be physically and psychologically injured by it. Her condition was believed to be worsened by returning to work directly after childbirth. Loudon captured this diagnostic trend with the following: "From a modern viewpoint, the nature and extent of puerperal insanity in the 19th century appears to be a complex mixture of myth and reality during a period when childbirth held many real and imagined terrors" (p. 78). Ultimately, these conditions signified another manifestation of the "disordering" of womanhood.

Hysteria

With the advent of the psychoanalytic era of the 1800s and 1900s, hysteria began to be diagnosed more commonly in both men and women. However, it was largely understood as a female condition resulting from trauma that could not be consciously processed (Tasca et al., 2012). Hysteria could take different iterations, including a more melancholic form, a biological form, and a physical symptom with psychological rather than biological causes. Freud contributed considerably in this area. He saw hysteria as leading to functional impairments that produced a secondary benefit enabling the patient to avoid the source of distress. Freud's theory of hysteria perpetuated notions of women as weak and melodramatic, creating a profile of the somewhat manipulative and possessed hysteric.

There were other figures who popularized the condition of hysteria. Franz Anton Mesmer (1734-1815) made this treatment into a social spectacle. He performed his treatment of moving the "animal magnetism" fluids within the body at live, sold-out shows (Porter, 2002). Austrian physician Josef Breuer (1824–1925) was also known for his work with hysteria, and served as a mentor to Freud. A number of his patients were from the special wards in the oldest asylum in France, the Salpêtrière; they included pregnant and poor young women, a number of whom had been sex workers (Chessler, 2005).

Treatment in that era included smelling salts to resituate women's wandering wombs, tracing back to Hippocrates's original model (Tasca et al., 2012). Also used in the treatment of hysteria was hypnotism, which was further developed by the French physicians Philippe Pinel (1745-1826), and Jean-Martin Charcot (1825–1893). Charcot was a neurologist who was also an inspiration to Freud. He attempted to establish that hysteria had genetic predispositions and developed in men even more than women. Similarly to Mesmer, Charcot cultivated professional patients who would demonstrate various stages of hysteria before audiences of physicians and at other public lectures (Showalter, 1995). In hindsight, these fits were often more performance than reality, and a performance of gender at that— the frenzied madwoman convulsing on command.

Hysteria in the Western world appeared to be frequently triggered by fear or trauma. It often began with uterine pain, leading into paroxysms resembling epileptic seizures, crying, anxiety, and depression (Smith-Rosenberg, 1972). These episodes could end with a restful sleep or trance-like state that could last for days (Showalter, 1995). Many physicians blamed the instability of puberty and other reproductive milestones. The British neurologist Horatio Bryan Donkin (1842–1927), however, saw social repression and associated sexual inhibitions as part of the cause.

In an article on women in the 19th century, Smith-Rosenberg (1972) portrayed the American iteration of hysteria as reflecting the frustration of middle- to upper-class women chafing under rigid gender socialization. Over the course of the 19th century, clinical etiology shifted from the wandering uterus and reproductive models to more genetic and neurological causes. It was not uncommon for physicians to perceive hysterical women as unruly and difficult patients who brought on their conditions by resisting passive social roles. Rather than underscoring their gender oppression, this model justified the assertion of the male physician's dominance and control, as well as the infantilization of the female patient. Freud did feel that women's restriction to domestic activities was a source of hysteria. However, he came to misconstrue the sexual abuse reported by his famous case of Dora as hysteria rather than reality (Showalter, 1995).

Problematic treatments were applied to hysteria among working-class men (Showalter, 1995). Like women, they were more likely to be diagnosed with this condition than wealthier men, revealing the class bias inherent in the diagnosis. In one mode of treatment, what was essentially electric shock torture was administered to shell-shocked veterans. The men had developed mutism after witnessing the trauma of war and were painfully electrified into speaking again. Toward the end of the 19th century, hysteria became a diagnosis reserved for what is labeled today as conversion disorder. Symptoms include the loss of sight, speech, movement, sensation, taste, smell, and other senses, without physical cause. Many providers would likely be surprised to learn the gendered history of a diagnosis still in use today.

Neurasthenia

Neurasthenia was a new condition of this era, traced to at least the early 1800s in England (Showalter, 1995). Symptoms included depressed mood, as well as blushing, dizziness, headaches, insomnia, and uterine irritation. Gender role and class expectations also influenced its prevalence, as it was diagnosed more among men who were overworked and particularly intelligent (Hirshbein, 2010). Hence, women with neurasthenia were distinguished from those with hysteria as being more "cooperative, ladylike and well-bred" (Showalter, 1995, p. 134). In the 1860s, the American neurologist George Miller Beard (1839–1883) ascribed neurasthenia to the effects of urbanization and industrialization. Women in this era had greater mental activity, which was believed to drain their mental fortitude. One of the few female physicians in the United States, Dr. Margaret Cleaves (1848–1917), even agreed with this perspective. In 1886, she wrote a paper on neurasthenia in the United States, having diagnosed it in herself. She ascribed her neurasthenia to her professional ambition and intense work life, which required various absences from work to recover.

A common treatment for neurasthenia was the "rest cure," often administered to women (Showalter, 1995). The rest cure appeared to do more harm than good by restricting the patient's activity and independence. Often strong-willed women were prescribed the rest cure (Ussher, 1991), and its effects have been likened to that of the solitary confinement of prisoners. The rest cure was depicted in the classic story by Charlotte Perkins Gilman, *The Yellow Wallpaper* (1892). In it, a woman was forbidden from working, due to the stress it was thought to cause, and was sequestered in a room with yellow wallpaper. She was eventually driven to madness by the very treatment intended to heal her. Apparently Gilman conceived the story to show her physician the error of his ways when he prescribed this treatment for her (Thraillkill, 2002). The *Yellow Wallpaper* became a key social protest against the sexist mental health treatment of women during this period.

Nymphomania

Nymphomania was another mental illness that was diagnosed among women in this era (Groneman, 1994). The sexologist Alfred Kinsey (1894–1956) famously offered a definition of a nymphomaniac as "someone who has more sex than you do" (Groneman, 2001, p. 90). Kinsey hinted at the social construction of such a condition and the lack of real medical legitimacy. The original concept of nymphomania was premised on gender expectations that women would be sexually passive. The causes put forth for nymphomania included an enlarged clitoris, diseases of the reproductive system, and an irregular menstrual cycle. Women who engaged in incestuous, adulterous, flirtatious, lesbian, or masturbatory sexual activity might also be deemed nymphomaniacs. Other "deviants" warranting this label were sex workers and young girls who expressed sexual desire. Even women with more libido than their husbands were diagnosed as nymphomaniacs.

In the Renaissance era, treatment of nymphomaniacs could include bleedings and herbs to achieve humoral balance (Groneman, 2001). In a severe case, a woman was bled over thirty times until she perished. The 19th century witnessed treatments that were as creative as they were horrific: vaginal swabs with caustic borax, cold enemas, and the applications of vaginal leeches. All forms of gynecological surgeries were mobilized: ovariectomy, hysterectomy, clitoridectomy, labiotomy. Again, gynecologists varied in their evaluation of the appropriateness of these procedures, from conviction in their success to total denunciation.

As might be expected, "hypersexual" men were regarded quite differently than their female counterparts. These men received the label of "satyriasis," as if their sexual behavior was dissimilar in origin or expression (Groneman, 1994). In contrast to nymphomania, satyriasis was much less commonly diagnosed and did not result in the genital mutilation that women endured. This gender disparity suggested diverging expectations of sexual behavior and desire (Hirshbein, 2010). In this manner, physicians enforced the passivity of women with diagnosis and scalpel.

The sexual anxieties of physicians could appear in their perceptions of, and dealings with, "seductive" patients (Groneman, 1994). Some of the few female physicians were paired with female patients with problematic sexual behavior or delusions (McGovern, 1981). In fact, the few female physicians trained in the late 19th century tended to be assigned to the lower-status work of treating female patients in asylums. Women's mental health symptoms were also understood to have gynecological origins that were more comfortably discussed and disclosed to women doctors, behind closed doors. Thus, female physicians and patients were largely segregated from male physicians and patients.

Anorexia

A brief discussion of anorexia and how it was historically gendered is warranted. While food refusal had early origins as a sign of religious devoutness in medieval

Europe, the problem resurfaced in the late 19th century. Anorexia was often seen as a way to display psychological distress and self-expression, albeit maladaptive (Tomes, 1990). Others argued it was mostly an expression of powerlessness. Victorian doctors sometimes viewed young women with anorexia as attempting to control their families (Showalter, 1995). It followed that treatment involved asserting their male authority over these patients. Ussher (1991) viewed anorexia as a manifestation of the expectations of female restraint of the Victorian era, particularly around eating. Thus food became a place where distress was manifested and communicated, and a sign of upper class status to deny it. Many of these gender themes linger in the causes and understanding of anorexia today.

Kleptomania

A final condition relevant to this discussion is that of kleptomania. In a review of the research on kleptomania, Murray (1992) identified the development of this notion in the nineteenth century. Kleptomania was understood as a compulsive behavior found in mostly middle- to upper-class women who pilfered insignificant items for which they had no real need. Like other feminized mental illnesses, this behavior was attributed to menstruation and postpartum changes in mental health. Treatment included gynecological surgery or other treatments assigned to women with mental illness. Even in the 20th century, psychoanalytic theories have described kleptomania as a symbolic shoplifting of phalluses and anal fixations. In kleptomania and the aforementioned conditions, we see a continued focus on the sexualization and gendering of mental illness among women.

20TH CENTURY

In the early 20th century, psychiatrists continued to focus on gender attributions of mental illness, although blame shifted from the genitals to sex hormones (Hirshbein, 2010). Women with psychosis were seen as having more aggressive, and thus masculine, sexual behavior. They were also perceived as having more masculine secondary sex characteristics, such as increased hair growth. Men with mental illness were perceived as having more passive and thus feminine sexual behavior, as well as more feminine secondary sex characteristics. These theories inevitably failed to garner any supporting evidence.

Mental illnesses were thought to manifest at the time of stressful developmental milestones for women, such as puberty, childbearing, and menopause, which led to the development of hormone treatments (Hirshbein, 2010). However, there were critics of these gynecological theories of women's mental illness among many female, and some male, physicians throughout this time (Hirshbein, 2010; McGovern, 1981). These treatments were found to have little effect and fell into disuse. However, a number of psychiatrists continued to use vaginal smears to track potential signs of mental illness in women into the 1940s.

Psychological assessments were developed in line with these theories of gender and mental illness. A key figure in the creation of psychological assessment, Lewis Terman, along with Catharine Cox Miles, created the Masculine-Feminine Test (Terry, 1999). The test was used to help identify adherence to gender roles by psychiatric patients. Men and women with psychosis were seen as deviating from gender norms, and the test was designed to assist with diagnosis (Hirshbein, 2010). Digging a bit deeper into the history of this measure only yields more troubling information. The Masculine-Feminine Test was used to study the sexual behavior of gay prisoners, many whom were incarcerated on charges of sodomy (Terry, 1999). The results were used to assert that homosexuality was psychologically unhealthy. In fact, many of the early psychological assessments were developed for problematic purposes, such as the substantiation of eugenics theories of race and gender (Mizock & Harkins, 2009).

In several essays from the 1920s and 1930s, Freud developed theories of women's mental illness (Ussher, 1991), such as gendered notions of penis envy as well as a sense of inferiority to men and self-hatred. He argued that women needed to accept an infant in place of a penis. These theories were contested by his former disciple Karen Horney (1885–1952), a German psychoanalyst. Horney is credited with establishing one of the preeminent theories of female psychology. She emphasized social factors and women's disenfranchised position in their intrapsychic composition. She likened penis envy to a symbol of male narcissism in psychoanalysis. To counterbalance the theory of penis envy, she argued that men envied women's ability to carry children. The psychoanalytic zeitgeist at this time continued to reflect women's subjugation in the broader culture. However, critics, often female, continued to question this misogynistic hegemony in the mental health field.

Psychiatric Hospitalization

Another development in mental health treatment that concerned women during this period was in the area of psychiatric hospitalizations. After World War II, psychiatric hospital admissions changed from mostly older men to younger, "neurotic" women (Hirshbein, 2006). Women were more likely to be featured in clinical trials of psychiatric medication, but this was not typically noted in the titles or abstracts of these research papers. Women were seen as more likely to have depression than men because of estrogen, and depressed men were thus administered testosterone. The effects of the social conditions and gender roles of women continued to be largely ignored.

In a relevant study, Braslow and Starks (2005) reviewed the psychiatric records from a hospital in California after World War II (1935–1960). They found an increase in hospitalization rates of patients without psychosis, and gender appeared to have a major influence on the process of admission, diagnosis, and treatment. This included the application of lobotomy to women at six times the rate of men, in spite of equivalent indications. They cited a larger investigation of lobotomy practices, which also found an imbalanced gender ratio of 60% women to 40% men (Kramer, 1954). At this hospital, women were administered antipsychotic drugs and electroconvulsive therapy (ECT) at disproportionate frequencies, a practice that was not unusual for this time (Braslow & Starks, 2005).

Physicians' notes suggest that women may have been administered ECT and lobotomy more often despite the risks, because physicians believed they needed their brains less (Ussher, 1991). Depressed housewives featured among lobotomy cases. Some physicians reasoned lobotomy would make them more effective in returning to the role of housewife, or able to cope with unhappy marriages (Showalter, 1995; Ussher, 1991). In Braslow and Starks's (2005) hospital records review, physicians' notes suggested that it was more acceptable for women to have a passive, childlike, and apathetic disposition than men following lobotomy. A docile woman would be less resistant to her domestic responsibilities and her relationship to her husband.

In contrast, some physicians interpreted the depression of men as stemming from unemployment and dominant wives (Braslow & Starks, 2005). After being discharged, men were expected to sustain ambition and motivation to succeed professionally, while maintaining financial independence and autonomy from the medical system. In the end, male and female patients alike were treated with antipsychotic medication, lobotomy, and ECT, even if they were not psychotic but were simply distressed by their gender roles. This made both men and women victims of gender biases of the 20th-century mental health system.

Sterilization

Sterilization is another misfortune of the mental institutions of that era. It is sometimes forgotten that people with SMI and intellectual disabilities were victims of the Holocaust in addition to Jews. Over 200,0000 psychiatric patients were murdered and more than 400,000 sterilized, not solely because they were considered unworthy of life, but also because it would cut health care costs (Torrey & Yolken, 2010). Some say the sterilization of these patients deviated from previous medical practice and violated the medical oath to "do no harm" (Braslow, 1996).

However, the converse appears to be true, as in many of the cases we have reviewed. In the United States people with SMI were commonly sterilized, reflecting physicians' purported social values. Eugenic beliefs infiltrated the medical system, and many physicians genuinely believed they were protecting the public from the genetic influence of mental illness. In an older medical record review, Braslow (1996) described the California state hospitals as contributing 50% to 80% to the national sterilization rate from the 1920s through the 1950s. These procedures were often performed without the consent of the patient's family.

Conversely, Tomes (1990) argued that many of the sterilization procedures performed in people with mental illness were done on men rather than women. In the particular state hospital Braslow (1996) researched, physicians erroneously documented reasons for vasectomies as producing an increase in hormones that would restore health to the mind and body. For female patients, sterilization was seen as preventing the stress of pregnancy and motherhood among women with mental illness—one of the primary complaints at admission (Braslow, 1996). Due to publicity about the Nazi sterilization practices, the sterilization of men and women in psychiatric hospitals diminished, but eugenic sterilization continued in certain states, peaking in the 1950s. It wasn't until as late as the 1970s that some state eugenics boards were finally disbanded (Schoen, 2001). In 1978 the Federal Sterilization Guidelines were passed to protect individuals from involuntary sterilization—recognized as a violation of civil and human rights. Laws and regulations such as these are in place today to better protect the welfare of women, and men, with mental illness in treatment facilities.

Antipsychiatry Movement

Problems in the treatment of people with mental illness, including that of women, continued from the 1920s through the 1960s. Showalter (1995) referred to this period as "psychiatric modernism" and highlighted the male-dominated nature of the antipsychiatry movement during this time. Antipsychiatry leaders critiqued the power imbalance in mainstream medicine and the harmful treatments many psychiatric patients endured as their rights were ignored. The antipsychiatry movement was inspired by the civil rights movements of the 1960s, but the leaders in the movement often overlooked women's issues. While one antipsychiatry leader, R. D. Laing, did see the impact of women's oppression on the mental health of some of his female patients, some believe he exploited his female patients for his own case studies.

Some followers of Laing even used radical politics to justify having sex with patients. As part of psychiatrist David Cooper's "bed therapy," he claimed to liberate women through orgasm that he himself would produce (Showalter, 1995). John Rosen was another American psychiatrist whose direct psychoanalysis approach included sexual acts, physical abuse, and humiliation (Ussher, 1991). It was not until the 1970s that awareness increased about sexual abuse of patients by providers. In the 1950s and 1960s, some psychoanalysts even married their patients, in what Chesler (2005) described as "psychological incest" (p. 22). Today, regional and national regulations prohibit such exploitations of gender by mental health providers, including the American Psychological Association's Ethics Code (2017). However, these ethical guidelines have not eliminated therapist abuse altogether, reflecting continuing problems with gender and power in women's mental health care.

CONCLUSION

It is easy to point a finger at historical injustices in mental health treatment using a "presentist" lens. However, recognizing the impact of gender bias on the history of mental health treatment of women illuminates contemporary gender issues that persist in treatment, along with the biological essentialism that is implicated in their causes. Women still face higher rates of mental health problems like depression. These disparities continue to be attributed to genetic and biological sex differences. Diagnoses like hysteria have been largely left behind in the Western world, but we face additions to the American Psychiatric Association's *Diagnostic and Statistical Manual of Mental Disorders* (DSM-5), such as "Premenstrual Dysphoric Disorder," that arguably pathologize female biology. In the end, feminist therapy brought the perspective of women's issues to mental health care, not antipsychiatry. In the following chapters, we will describe more of the implications of feminist and gender-sensitive psychotherapy for women with SMI and provide some case examples to bring to life gender issues in the mental health experiences of women with SMI today.

DISCUSSION QUESTIONS

1. How do you think the history of mental health treatment of women affects perceptions of women with SMI today? Is history repeating itself? In what ways do you feel we have made progress or continue to be stuck in past gender biases of mental illness?
2. What are some of the potential benefits and disadvantages of biomedical understandings of gender differences in SMI? How have these changed or stayed the same over time, and what can be learned from this history?
3. What needs to change in the contemporary approach to the treatment of women with SMI? What changes do you feel need to be made in public policy and government to better meet the needs of women with SMI?

ACTIVITIES

1. *History lesson.* Select one of the past treatments (e.g., clitoridectomy, ovariectomy, female sterilization, lobotomy, smelling salts, rest cure, asylum "laundry therapy") or historically bound afflictions (e.g., hysteria, puerperal/reflex/lactational insanity, nymphomania, kleptomania) commonly assigned to women. Conduct additional research about this treatment or condition. Collect at least four facts for each topic and share them with a group if available. Relate these practices and conditions to perspectives on gender at that time.
2. *DSM-5 diagnoses.* Identify a DSM-5 diagnosis that might increase stigma of women's mental health (e.g., Premenstrual Dysphoric Disorder, Anorexia/Bulimia, Borderline Personality Disorder, Histrionic Personality Disorder, Dependent Personality Disorder). Then do one of the following and provide your rationale: (a) propose

reasons for removing the diagnosis; (b) propose reasons for revising the diagnostic criteria; or (c) propose an alternative diagnosis to reduce gender bias. Discuss (possibly in a group) how these diagnostic changes can be compared and contrasted, identifying themes in the use of language, implicit attitudes about gender, and types of revisions that are needed.

3

Women with Serious Mental Illness, Resilience, and the Recovery Movement

Imagine you are severely depressed, wondering if there is any purpose to life, and having difficulty differentiating reality. You are taken to an institution where they lock you away from your loved ones, and provide treatments that only make you more depressed and scared. To add to this, a spouse or provider could decide to keep you there indeterminably. This has been the case for many women who have been retraumatized by their treatment experiences.

Over time, things have gotten somewhat better in our mental health system. Women have demonstrated their resilience and used their voice to speak out about the egregiousness of mental health service delivery and the marginalization of people with serious mental illness (SMI). In the recovery movement of the 1970s (also known as the consumer movement), people with SMI advocated for their rights after having been released from institutions (Davidson & Roe, 2007). They called themselves ex-patients, consumers, or survivors, and advocated for their right to be treated as more than just a mental health problem. These ex-patients became leaders in mental health policy reform.

Alongside this movement, the World Health Organization conducted research that found partial to full capacity for recovery among 25% to 65% of people with SMI, challenging societal and clinical beliefs that patients are doomed to a life as a "mental patient" (Carpenter & Kirkpatrick, 1988; World Health Organization, 1973). This research led to the realization that a mental illness was not necessarily a permanent experience that could take over one's life. This was at odds with the hopeless prognoses assigned to many people who had been institutionalized for most of their life (Davidson & Roe, 2007).

WHAT DOES RECOVERY MEAN?

In contrast to how the term has been historically used in the substance abuse field, recovery in the mental health field has come to mean recovery beyond the effects of having a mental illness (Davidson & White, 2007). It does not necessarily signify a resolution or elimination of all symptoms. Rather, it can refer to recovery from a life of stigma, marginalization, and oppression. From this standpoint, recovery means that a mental health challenge is only one aspect in the life of an individual with many assets, strengths, capabilities, and interests. People in recovery are viewed as having a desire for self-determination and the right to live a life of meaning as they so define (Davidson et al., 2009).

As people have engaged in these advocacy efforts, systems have become more invested in this shift in how mental health services are delivered. Recovery-oriented care has become the recommendation of the President's New Freedom Commission on Mental Health (U.S. Department of Health and Human Services, 2003) and the Federal Action Agenda (Department of Health and Human Services, 2005). In 2003, President George W. Bush mandated this philosophy of care for the provision of mental health services in the United States. This change in national policy reflects increasing investment in the recovery process in psychiatric settings around the world.

Foundations of recovery conceptualize experiences of stigma and marginalization as rampant among those with SMI. The experiences of individuals may be as much about the effects of marginalization as the symptoms of mental illness itself (Anthony, 1993; Davidson, 2009). Leaders in the recovery movement put forth that all people with SMI have strengths and capabilities, and that everyone should be able to live a life of meaning.

Tondora and colleagues (2008) conducted research on the personal dimensions of recovery. They identified internal factors (insight, resilience, determination, self-managed care, empowerment) and external factors (peer support, social support, family). The following qualitative themes have also emerged from personal narratives of recovery:

- Reawakening of hope after despair
- Moving from withdrawal to engagement and active participation in life
- Active coping rather than passive adjustment
- Moving from alienation to a sense of meaning and purpose
- A complex and nonlinear journey
- Thriving, not just surviving
- No longer seeing oneself as a person primarily with a psychiatric disorder and reclaiming a positive sense of self.

The Substance Abuse and Mental Health Services Administration (SAMSHA, 2008) developed a National Consensus Statement on Recovery that identified the 10 Fundamental Components of Recovery. These components indicate that recovery is self-directed, individualized, empowering, holistic, nonlinear, strengths-based, peer-supported, and respectful, and instills both responsibility and hope. The idea is that these constructs of recovery can help individuals build a meaningful life beyond the effects of mental illness as they strive to achieve their potential and personal goals.

As one can imagine, a recovery-oriented care service delivery model has important implications for women. As we look back at the history of women in the mental health system and ongoing concerns with oppression, it only makes sense that transformation of mental health systems to recovery-oriented care could make an immense impact on the lives of women with SMI. Hence, the basic components of recovery-oriented care will be explored in the next section of this chapter.

THE 10 FUNDAMENTAL COMPONENTS OF RECOVERY

Experiencing Support from Others

The value of providing and experiencing support from others is multifold. Many times those with SMI have been isolated or separated from family, romantic partnerships, and meaningful relationships in the community. The stigma and marginalization that is a part of the experience of mental illness is disenfranchising. To be cast out and unaccepted by one's community without core social support can in itself be debilitating. In Western culture the tradition is to offer inpatient and sometimes long-term hospitalization (Khandelwal, Jhingan, Ramesh, Gupta, & Srivastava, 2004). In contrast, many Eastern cultural traditions may keep people with SMI at home, in their community, or find other ways to incorporate them into daily life, such as by finding a place for them in their workspace (Jablensky et al., 1992). The World Health Organization has also found better outcomes in some studies of those in developing countries, where individuals are more typically cared for by their families and community members (Jablensky et al., 1992).

Relatedly, one of the most important elements of evidence-based treatment for those with SMI is family support and involvement, as highlighted by the Schizophrenia Patient Outcomes Research Team study (Dixon et al., 2009). Family psychoeducation has also been shown to consistently improve outcomes for people in recovery and caregivers (Dixon et al., 2001).

Experiencing support from others can also have multiple definitions, and support not necessarily have to come from one's family of origin. Support can come from a range of community members such as a spiritual leader, mentor, job coach, coworker, case manager, or peer. Recovery is not a process that can be done alone (Davidson et al., 2005). It is crucial for people in recovery to feel part of a community, and to have supportive individuals in their lives who provide encouragement and support throughout times of challenge and wellness.

Renewal of Hope and Commitment

In the process of recovery, hope is fundamental. This is the possibility for a renewed sense of purpose and self. Belief in the person with SMI can offer important sources of hope (Davidson et al., 2005). Hope can renew motivation and desire and contribute to the recovery process. In this vein, recovery also means that individuals can feel capable of expanding their personal abilities and make their own choices, regardless of the state of their illness or symptoms (Resnick, Rosenheck, & Lehman, 2004). In many studies hope has been correlated strongly with well-being, quality of life, spirituality, resiliency, self-esteem, self-confidence, self-transcendence, and subjective global life satisfaction (Corrigan, McCorkle, Schell, & Kidder, 2003; Davis, 2005; Landeen, Pawlick, Woodside, Kirkpatrick, & Byrne, 2000; Phillips-Salimi, Haase, Kintner, Monahan, & Azzouz, 2007; Wahl et al., 2004).

The values of hope and commitment hold particular meaning for women with SMI. Hope and belief in the individual confront challenges that may face women with SMI who are experiencing intersecting oppressive experiences of psychiatric stigma and sexism or misogyny. Housing can also foster hope and recovery among women with SMI, as shown in at least two different studies (Kirst, Zerger, Harris, Plenert, & Stergiopoulos, 2014; Manuel, Hinterland, Conover, & Herman, 2012). The recovery literature indicates that among women with SMI, having social connections that are reciprocal and fulfilling can motivate them to get out of the hospital and have hope for their success (Manuel et al., 2012).

Meaningful Activities or Valued Social Roles

The importance of positive activities in life and valued social roles should not be underestimated. People with SMI can feel cut off from society and the full rights of citizenship (Rowe, 2015). Being able to engage in functional social roles such as employee, student, friend, or even voter is central to recovery (Davidson et al., 2005).

Many women have found that the SMI has led to a change in the traditional roles they might have held (Chernomas, Clarke, & Chisholm, 2000). This can have a particular impact as women may be socialized to become mothers or caregivers or to play other important roles within families and relationships that are then limited by an SMI. It is important that women with SMI are allowed to expand their social roles and associated value in society.

Redefinition of Self

Redefinition of the self is one of the most consistent constructs that appears in the recovery literature. This relates to seeing oneself not as a mental health patient, but as an individual with strengths, aspirations, capabilities, and responsibilities, with a right to live one's life as desired. In essence, this perception of the self rejects the sociopolitical context frequently projected on those with mental illness. This concept portrays identity as multidimensional—that being a mental health patient does not define oneself (Davidson et al., 2005). This is tremendously important, as many people have been given a negative prognosis that their life will become solely focused on taking medications, going to therapy, receiving disability income, and obtaining supportive housing (Copeland, 2007). This shocking life sentence can do great harm, increase internalized stigma, and diminish self-worth. People with SMI can thus be robbed of a belief in their own capacity to heal and recover, and the motivation to pursue their life goals.

The recovery concept of a redefinition of the self holds particular value for women with SMI who have faced stigma that has interfered with their life goals (Wisdom, Bruce, Saedi, Weis, & Green, 2008). These goals may be related to career or family aspirations. Allowing these women to redefine themselves in a way that provides purpose and meaning can promote healing and rebirth.

Management of Symptoms

Complete recovery from symptoms may not be a goal; it may not be expected, or even necessary. Rather, recovery represents the capacity to manage symptoms in a way that works for the individual (Davidson et al., 2005). This perspective acknowledges that there will be periods that are more challenging and difficult, but there will be other periods where one may be symptom-free or have an increased capacity to deal with symptoms. The entire journey is part of the nonlinear recovery process. Individuals are empowered to engage in methods that help them with symptoms as they choose, rather than being a passive recipient of services who is told what to do or how to deal with symptoms.

Women with SMI have talked about the value of being able to deal with their symptoms in a way that makes sense for them and their life (Manuel et al., 2012). They have also stated that when symptoms reemerge, say after a hospitalization, it is important to have a lot of support from providers. This support might mean being able to phone someone when symptoms reappear and having social connections who can help. Women with SMI have also discussed the value of taking responsibility for doing things to help manage symptoms, such as taking medications, engaging in treatment, attending appointments and programs, and avoiding social isolation. Having access to appropriate mental health care is invaluable for maintaining wellness, according to women with SMI. The recovery perspective involves shifting from an illness narrative to a strengths-based approach, as suggested by the *Recovery to Practice Curriculum* (APA & Jansen, 2014).

Empowerment and Engagement in Full Rights of Citizenship

There are different levels of citizenship: non-citizenship, in which an individual is separated from society; second-class citizenship, in which an individual has suboptimal connections to society; or full citizenship, in which an individual has strong ties to systems, rights, and responsibilities (Rowe, 1999). Full citizenship involves valued social roles, responsibilities, and resources (Ponce & Rowe, 2018). People with SMI and other life disruptions such as addiction, homelessness, or criminal justice involvement have the right to full citizenship, but instead they frequently experience non-citizenship, stigma, and marginalization. People in recovery can demand their full rights to citizenship, such as the right to decide where to live, how to spend their time, and whom to love. They can be empowered to engage in and take on responsibilities like other citizens do, such as having a job, voting, or community organizing (Davidson et al., 2005).

Rapp and Goscha (2012) explained how the social processes and practices contribute to oppressive experiences for people with mental illness. They advocated for a focus and shift toward maximizing human potential and well-being, with movement into the community rather than withdrawal from it. This focus can become a transformative process rather than a focus on barriers. As the Rev. Dr. Martin Luther King, Jr. said, "Whatever affects one directly affects all indirectly. I can never be what I ought to be until you are what you ought to be. This is the interrelated structure of society" (King, 1967, p. 1).

Recovery narratives of women with SMI also reflect their desire to be a part of society (Manuel et al., 2012). They have voiced how the stigma of mental illness and being shunned can lead to social isolation, making them feel treated like they are contagious. The ability to reengage in society and have a connection to others as a friend, mother, coworker, or family member is crucial to their successful transition into the community from a hospital setting.

Assuming Control and Agency

Imagine being told that you must take a specific medication every day, that you need to live in a certain area of town with people you do not know, and that you need to check in for appointments at a local mental health center every week. To remain in your supportive housing, you have to attend a specific number of therapy groups every week. At least once a month you are expected to have your blood drawn to see how your medication is affecting your body. You must be agreeable to medication changes, despite the complicated side effects you experience. Meanwhile, you would like to attend some classes at the local university on finances and get a part-time job to earn money and feel engaged with other people on a regular basis. You would also like the time and space to try to date a bit on the weekend. However, it is difficult to fit everything in your life with so many expectations from your providers to manage your symptoms and keep you out of the hospital.

This is all too often the life that is prescribed for people with SMI. No wonder the concepts of assuming control and agency in one's life hold great importance! Many times, those with SMI feel like they have a loss of control, with many of their rights taken away. They may have been hospitalized against their will, medicated against their wishes, detained, arrested, and tasered. A judge may have appointed a conservator to make decisions about their welfare, their finances, and their medical treatment. Not surprisingly, women with SMI have emphasized the importance of having autonomy and agency in relation to support from others and specifically from treatment supports (Manuel et al., 2012). Women with SMI have highlighted the value of support—but a type that honors their perspective and voice. After experiencing the loss of basic human rights and often the lack of full citizenship, being able to assume control and agency in one's life may serve as a major impetus toward recovery.

Acknowledgment and Understanding of Illness and Self-Direction

This recovery concept entails that individuals acknowledge and accept the limitations they experience as a result of their mental illness. This can help them unearth their talents, strengths, and new possibilities that will empower them to reach their personal life goals even with a disability (Davidson et al., 2005). This does not mean they must accept that they have a specific mental illness. Rather, they recognize they have some challenges and build increased understanding for how they are going to use their own capabilities and strengths to pursue life goals. A qualitative study among women with serious depression highlighted the theme of taking one's own responsibility for wellness, admitting when one needs help, and learning to cope (Snell-Rod et al., 2017). In this study, the women discussed that attending treatment services only goes so far and that individuals are the ones who must put things into action to make changes in their lives and start feeling better. Although support can come from treatment services, they also valued self-sufficiency.

Systems are encouraged to shift away from just treating or rehabilitating people toward supporting people in their own efforts to manage and overcome specific mental health challenges, while they take their own paths and own their own responsibility for working toward their goals and life dreams (Davidson et al., 2007). People with SMI can become the drivers of their own recovery experience rather than being told how their life will be and what they should do as "mental patients." This shift from a traditional approach to a self-directed one increases transparency, flexibility , and collaboration in care between providers and the recipients of care (APA & Jansen, 2014). Assertive community treatment, supported employment, cognitive-behavioral therapy, skills training, and other evidence-based treatments could help women to take responsibility for their clinical care at a mental health organization (Dixon et al., 2009).

RECOVERY PROGRAMMING FOR WOMEN

As we consider these basic components of recovery, our thinking may shift with regard to how people experience their mental health challenges and the messages in this experience. A traditional, illness-based model might be reflected by a statement like this: "I have been told I have this serious diagnosis called schizophrenia, which means I have to take medications daily, apply for disability income, and make treatment my primary focus. I cannot pursue my college education and the work I desire." A more hopeful message is, "Yes, I have this challenge, but these are the ways I am finding to deal with it. Here is how you can partner with me in those endeavors." What a transformation! Unfortunately, the first message is the one that many people receive. It's no wonder many people refuse to accept a diagnosis that involves giving up their dreams and hopes for the future. Ultimately, as providers partner with people in recovery, there is a movement away from concepts like compliance, imposing treatments rather than just offering them. There is a change from controlling or compulsion to understanding that the woman in recovery is the expert in her care (Slade, 2009).

A recovery perspective can have an amazing impact on the experiences of women in recovery and can serve as a guide for great transformations in our mental health systems. Even today, treatment of women in the mental health system can be uncomfortable, sexist, and traumatic (Frueh et al., 2005). A shift to a recovery-oriented model can lead to empirical improvements and reported qualitative improvements.

Systemic reviews indicate the need for more empirical research focused on the impact of recovery-oriented care, though there is some literature that suggests there may be an improvement in quality of life for people in recovery, better engagement in treatment, and fewer social problems (Guidjonsson et al., 2011; Kidd, McKenzie, & Virdie, 2014). Qualitative research has demonstrated the beneficial effects of implementation of four factors of the recovery orientation (Mancini, 2007): meaningful activities, supportive professional relationships, peer support, and choice of preferred treatment options, which is associated with an increase in self-efficacy. Other studies indicate that this model can help providers improve their attitudes toward those in recovery, increase their knowledge base, and improve their clinical practice (Kidd et al., 2014). Staff education in the recovery perspective has also been shown to have a positive impact on client functioning (Elbaz-Haddad & Savaya, 2011).

Interestingly, an increase in privacy on inpatient psychiatric units, which aligns with recovery-oriented practice, leads to a higher likelihood that individuals will choose to take their medications (Frueh et al., 2005). Settings that incorporate women's preferences for personal space can have a positive impact on their decisions to take medications or not. Such conceptual shifts in understanding seem like small alterations, but they can make a big difference in how a woman experiences treatment and her options of choice and control in such a milieu.

BIOLOGICAL AND DEVELOPMENTAL CONCERNS
AMONG WOMEN WITH SMI

Women's engagement in their recovery journey should be person-centered and shaped by their uniqueness, meaning not only their choices and goals, but also their biological and developmental experiences. Thus, the literature should reflect the specific experiences of women in this area in order to be integrated into a cohesive and effective approach in care for each woman. In this section, issues pertaining to the biological and developmental concerns of women with SMI will be addressed with regard to medications, reproductive issues, general physical well-being, and life expectancy.

Medications

The literature indicates that women and men may respond differently to psychotropic medications. However, attention is not always paid to this issue, an oversight that could be of serious concern. For instance, responses to antipsychotic use among women and men are related to gender-specific factors such as smoking, concurrent medications, exercise, substance use, hormonal transitions, body build, and diet (Seeman, 2004). Women may need a smaller dosage of an antipsychotic medication than men to reach the same effect. Nonetheless, antipsychotic prescription guidelines do not make this gender differentiation (Anthony & Berg, 2002; Anthony & Berg, 2002a; Harris, Benet, & Schwartz, 1995; Kashuba & Nafziger, 1998). Women's bodies typically have 25% more adipose tissue, and since most antipsychotic drugs accumulate in lipid stores, this makes a difference in terms of how the drug is metabolized and its effectiveness (Beierle, Meibohm, & Derendorf, 1999). Since women have more adipose tissue, more of the antipsychotics accumulate over time in the body, a factor that should be considered when women are given depot injections (Seeman, 2004). The literature indicates that after stabilization with a particular depot injection, intervals between doses of the injection should be longer for women than for men (Altamura et al., 2003; Daniel, 2003).

Women with schizophrenia are also more likely than their male counterparts to be taking adjunct drugs. Hence, there is increased opportunity for drug interactions, which can either lower or raise antipsychotic serum levels. Levels can also be affected by factors such as smoking, alcohol intake, and coffee consumption (Balant-Gorgia, Gex-Fabry, & Balant, 1996; Gex-Fabry, Balant-Gorgia, & Balant, 2001).

Other literature in this area points to factors such as acute dystonia, which occurred more often in one sample of women than men with first-episode psychosis, even though this has been thought to be more common among men (Casey, 1991). Though men and women may have similar adverse drug effects, those among women have been more serious (Miller, 2001). Due to the effects of antipsychotics, women also need mammograms, electrocardiograms, bone density scans, diabetes and cardiovascular workups, as well as dosage modulation for aging women (Seeman, 2004). Women need bone density scans due to the effect of low estrogen levels and an increase in prolactin due to antipsychotics, which can lead to osteoporosis or bone breakage (Becker et al., 2003; Wieck & Haddad, 2003). There is some concern that the higher prolactin levels may put women at increased risk for breast cancer. Dosage modulation in older women is important because renal excretion becomes progressively impaired as people age and drugs do not metabolize as quickly (Seeman, 2004).

As women are more likely than men to have adverse weight gain related to antipsychotics, they should be evaluated for weight gain regularly, especially given research showing that women are more concerned than men about obesity. This pertains to the impact of obesity on self-image in an appearance-focused society (Allison et al., 1999; Homel, Casey, & Allison, 2002). Ideally, prescribers would discuss healthy weight and contributing factors (diet, exercise, smoking) at the initial assessment so that wellness goals could be maintained and monitored from a proactive standpoint.

Hormonal Factors

Though we know hormones play a role in how women may experience mood and mental illness, there is little research in this area on women with SMI (Seeman, 2004). During pregnancy, the postpartum period, and menopause, assessment for prescription changes may be needed, such as possible dosage modulations. Hormonal fluctuations during the menstrual cycle could affect different systems of the body and impact protein binding and the volume of distribution of drugs, requiring variations in prescribing (Kashuba & Nafziger, 1998; Seeman, 2004).

The literature also indicates that women experience different side effects than men, such as drug-induced hyperprolactinemia when taking antipsychotics (Kuruvilla, Peedicavil, Srikrishna, Kuruvilla, & Kanagasa-Bapathy, 1992; Naidoo, Kinion, Gilmore, Liu, & Halbreich, 2003). Prolactin levels increase up to 10 times normal with this medication, resulting in rates of amenorrhea as high as 78% (Wieck & Haddad, 2003).

Though there is some literature to support the concept that women have a better response to antipsychotic treatment than men, this may have to do with many other variables and less to do with the response to medication. Instead, this difference may be related to women's lifestyle differences, enhanced social support, and relative hormonal protection (Meltzer et al., 1997; Seeman, 2004; Torgalsboen, 1999). However, the concept that needs to be considered more widely is that if women happen to have better outcomes, then their mainte-nance antipsychotic doses could be less than in men (Seeman, 2004). There is also some question about the need to stay on medications for a lifetime, which is frequently the default position despite the considerable effects from lifetime use of medications. Moreover, there is some evidence that individuals may do better if they only have episodic pharmacologic treatment (Omachi & Sumiyoshi, 2018; Thompson, Singh, & Birchwood, 2016).

Pregnancy and Breastfeeding

There should be increased knowledge and focus on pregnant women with SMI in relation to the effect of drugs on labor, developmental challenges, and potential effects of withdrawal for the infant and behavioral toxicity (American Academy of Pediatrics Committee on Drugs, 2000; Boyle, 2002; Craig & Abel, 2001; Dawes & Chowienczyk, 2001; Ernst & Goldberg, 2002; Frederikson, 2001; Giere, 2001; Patton, Misri, Corral, Perry, & Kuan, 2002; Seeman, 2004; Shehata & Nelson-Piercy, 2001; Winans, 2001; Wyska & Jusko, 2001). For instance, due to hormonal changes, women may need less of a drug during pregnancy than when they are not pregnant (Seeman, 2004).

Breastfeeding has to be conceptualized differently as well, since medications that may be safe to take during pregnancy may not be safe during breastfeeding. According to some recommendations, it may be best to refrain from taking medications while nursing (Della-Giustina & Chow, 2003). Ascertaining whether medication is needed and then choosing the safest medication is a wise approach. If medication is needed, the drug chosen should have a low milk-to-plasma ratio, a high molecular weight, a short half-life, and high protein binding in maternal serum; it should be ionized in maternal plasma and should be non-lipophilic. If there is a chance that a medication could put the infant at risk, the infant should be monitored for drug levels. It is also suggested that a mother take her medication after she has completed a breastfeeding session, or before the baby's longest sleep period of the day. This can limit the baby's exposure to the medication.

Recent research shows women are more likely to have serious concerns with postpartum depression if they have particularly painful healing periods after giving birth. However, rarely do they experience postpartum care that is as good as their prenatal care, which might be able to prevent more serious postpartum mental health issues (Ou, Zhou, & Xiang, 2018). Longitudinal studies suggest that recovering from giving birth involves much more than the healing of the reproductive system (McGovern et al., 2006). There is a significant risk of depression during pregnancy, ranging from 7% to 26% (Hobfoll, Ritter, Lavin, Hulsizer, & Cameron, 1995). Depression during pregnancy is a predictor of postpartum depression (Graff, Dyck, & Schallow, 1991). The incidence of postpartum depression is 10% to 15% in all women; it affects the mother's functioning and ability to care for the infant and interrupts the functioning of relationships (Graff et al., 1991; Logsdon, Wisner, Billings, & Shanahan, 2006; Moses-Kolko, & Roth, 2004).

Unfortunately, the likelihood that women will receive mental health treatment for postpartum depression is not high given that many physicians do not regularly screen for it, refer women for treatment, or have the ability to do so. Addressing such challenges and barriers is crucial to ensuring that women receive the appropriate mental health treatment throughout their maternal care (Logsdon et al.,

2006). The peripartum period may be even more challenging for women already diagnosed with SMI as they may have intersecting challenges that can make the experience even more difficult (Mowbray, Oyserman, Bybee, MacFarlane, & Rueda-Riedle, 2001).

Physical Well-Being and Life Expectancy

Individuals with SMI have an increased risk of comorbid physical conditions and a much lower life expectancy than those without SMI (Druss et al., 2018; Miller, Paschall, & Svendsen, 2006). In fact, standardized mortality ratios among psychiatric patients are more than twice those of the general population, and life expectancy is 25 to 30 years less than the general population (Colton & Manderscheid, 2006; DeHert et al., 2011; Felker, Yazel, & Short, 1996). A more recent study has indicated that obesity, hypertension, diabetes, and chronic obstructive pulmonary disease are the most prevalent comorbidities among those with SMI (Miller et al., 2006). Potential factors include poor hygiene, reduced physical activity, a high rate of smoking, substance use, medication-induced weight gain, and poor social support, all of which likely contribute to these physical challenges. Women are at an increased risk of more life-years lost than men (Chang et al., 2011). Men with schizophrenia and women with schizoaffective disorders are at the highest end of life-years lost. Many of the experiences that contribute to the life-years lost relate to smoking, diabetes, and obesity, which are preventable causes of premature death.

The data indicate that greater attention and focus on exercise can be beneficial to those with SMI, using an aerobic and resistance training model (Marzolini, Jensen, & Melville, 2009). Women with schizophrenia are less likely to exercise than men on a weekly basis (Brown, Birtwistle, Roe, & Thompson, 1999). An exercise program has been associated with significant improvements in overall mental health and depressive symptoms, improvement in functional exercise capacity, and muscular strength. Interestingly, reduction in depressive symptoms was also related to a greater likelihood to exercise.

Clearly, recovery-oriented care must take into account the unique biological and developmental concerns for women with SMI. In the next section, several case narratives will depict some of the unique experiences of women with SMI, including biological and developmental concerns. The recovery-oriented model will be applied to their stories to highlight this perspective, as well as clinical strategies for enhancing empowerment in their mental health care.

CASE NARRATIVES

Case 1: Savannah

"Savannah" is a White, American, 32-year-old woman who experienced her first psychotic break at age 26. She hears voices and believes that computers installed a pacemaker in her body while she slept. She believes that computers have taken over the world and that she must find and throw away computers and related technology so humans can regain their power. These beliefs have led her to take computers from her family members and destroy them by dropping them, running them over with a car, or lighting them on fire. When she is around a computer she becomes agitated and explains that people working on the computers need to get out from under their control.

Savannah has a master's degree in business. She was working in business administration when she experienced a psychotic break. Her aunt helped her take a medical leave during this time so she could try to hold on to her job. However, when she returned to work after her first hospitalization, she stopped taking her medications due to excruciating akathisia, weight gain, and the development of diabetes. She threw three computers out of the window at work, resulting in her job loss.

Savannah's aunt helped her get support again through the mental health system. She was restarted on a different antipsychotic with preventive treatment for side effects, since she felt she would rather die than have akathisia again or keep gaining weight. Some of the initial challenges she faced were increased agitation from her delusional beliefs during certain parts of her menstrual cycle; at other times she experienced increased positive results from the medications. Her providers noticed and tracked the cyclical patterns of her mood and psychotic symptoms, providing different pharmacologic interventions during these times. She worked with recovery-oriented clinicians who enabled her to communicate her desires and experiences of the medications, while they offered their expertise to best inform the decision-making process. Savannah included the support of her aunt, her grandfather, and a best friend in this collaborative process.

Some of the recovery-oriented nature of Savannah's treatment included open communication practices, person-centered treatment planning, and increasing her experience of autonomy in an experience that initially felt involuntary since she had first been hospitalized against her will. Related to the challenges with weight gain and diabetes, in addition to alterations in prescribing, the psychiatrist, Savannah, and her clinician focused on wellness strategies. They developed a holistic plan including her preferred forms of exercise, such as weekend hiking, walking, and yoga one day a week, as well as different mechanisms to maintain a healthy diet. This plan helped her with mood, management of weight gain, and dealing with distress from psychotic symptoms.

The first few years after Savannah's psychotic break were rough. In time, she accepted that she had an illness and could recognize her challenges, enabling her to assume greater control and agency in her own life. She could then accept responsibility for communicating with her providers and natural supports about her mental health care and life goals. She set a goal to return to work because working brought meaning to her life. Her team supported this goal and adjusted her appointments, expectations, and pharmacologic regimen so that she could reengage with the world of work.

Soon Savannah found a new job and started working part-time with the plan to assume a full-time position within a year if she felt like things were going well. This endeavor was one of the most important parts of her recovery journey as it helped her embrace her identity and realize that she had every right to hope and believe that she could live a meaningful life. Savannah realized she had to do some things differently than before, such as drink much less alcohol and refrain from her occasional marijuana use as she realized it made her symptoms worse. She decided to get better sleep, watch her stress levels, and do things she enjoyed, such as spending time with friends, reading, playing the guitar, and cooking. She also realized that engaging in activities like these helped her keep her mind off thoughts about computers that were distressing. Savannah worked with a therapist over time about how to navigate her way in a world full of computers and technology, differentiating real threats from thoughts that she was in danger. This discernment helped her return to the business world where computers were a part of life, and she could come to tolerate them with more ease.

Case 2: Jennifer

"Jennifer," an outpatient psychotherapy client, is an African American woman who had just reached her 50th birthday when she faced a tragedy: Her 19-year-old son was unjustly killed by police in a protest about the profiling of young Black men. After he was shot, the police realized he was unarmed. The whole community mourned this loss. There was strong discord between this community and local law enforcement over racial profiling and injustices in the nation.

This experience was so traumatic for Jennifer that she could not speak for a month and barely ate. She lost 30 pounds in one month and her whole family grew concerned for her welfare. This occurred in the aftermath of episodes of severe depression throughout her life and four suicide attempts, two of which were very serious. Despite this history, Jennifer had been doing quite well for the past five years. She was working full-time, had raised her other son mostly on her own (he was currently living with her), and was dating a new man she felt she could trust. She was also consistently attending psychotherapy appointments and used therapy to process difficult emotional issues and to maintain wellness in her recovery journey.

Jennifer's parents and brother held a family discussion and decided they would ask her if it would be a good time to get some extra support or think about engaging in a crisis respite stabilization service program. This program is an alternative to a full psychiatric hospitalization, consisting of a temporary residential stay where mental health services are available and patients can typically come and go as they please. Jennifer was thankful that her family did not become overly intrusive or jump to the conclusion that she was suicidal and needed further intervention. In the past, she had had traumatizing experiences with involuntary hospitalizations. However, she was eventually able to discuss her emotional state with her family and began to strategize her care in the wake of this recent traumatic event.

Jennifer did not agree to go to crisis respite center, but initiated more sessions with her therapist, began attending a bereavement support group, and engaged in activism over the next few years. Jennifer also realized she had been working on a lifetime of recovery strategies that she could currently employ, such as spending time with her friends and family, seeking out spiritual guidance, engaging in pleasant hobbies such as listening to music and sewing dresses, and attending exercise classes. She reconnected with these recovery strategies, which served as forms of personal medicine and served as ways she could discharge some of her emotional distress. She communicated with her family about her need for space to process her grief and pain without being infantilized. In essence, Jennifer advocated for her right to have her own agency, autonomy, and personal control in a situation in which she lacked control with the loss of her son. Her family respected these wishes but also communicated about how they could check in with her in a reasonable way so she could access their support as needed.

Jennifer was going through menopause and felt like her hormonal shifts might be worsening her grief and the likelihood of a new depressive stage. She discussed this with her psychiatrist and explored pharmacologic strategies and physical interventions. The psychiatrist assessed her hormone levels and tracked how they affected her mood. She integrated some of her coping strategies into this process, which helped when she felt more depressed and had stronger feelings of grief.

One of the most meaningful recovery tools Jennifer used was getting more involved in the valued social role of community action and advocacy. Jennifer felt strongly about wanting to honor her son's memory with how she lived her life after he passed and served as an advocate in her local community related to the issues of racial profiling of young Black men. Jennifer felt a sense of empowerment by being involved in social justice action; she felt like she was making a difference in the world. Her story also highlights the sociocultural contributors to SMI for women, including experiences of racial violence and oppression.

CLINICAL APPLICATIONS

There are many clinical applications of a recovery perspective. Providers can take an egalitarian approach with women with SMI. This involves valuing the expertise of the individual in her own experience. The provider can be a partner in making decisions, setting goals, and planning treatment. It is important to take off the "expert hat" as someone with all of the answers, while retaining the capacity to offer whatever clinical expertise one can.

Person-centered treatment planning and shared decision-making models offer useful tools for implementing a recovery approach (Drake, Deegan, & Rapp, 2010; Tondora, Miller, Slade, & Davidson, 2014). A multicultural feminist framework can help to understand problems that arise from sociopolitical experiences of oppression toward women with SMI. This perspective highlights the experiences of stigma from mental illness and related intersections with racism, sexism, homophobia, and classism (Worell & Remer, 2003). It is important for providers to create a supportive, safe, and empowering spaces where women can be heard. This can validate their experiences and allow them to grow, heal, and use their own voices to decide what their recovery looks like.

When working with women in recovery to build hope, it is important for providers to listen nonjudgmentally and with trust and acceptance, believing in the women's potential and strength (Slade, 2009). Any setbacks can be viewed as part of the recovery process. Therapists can provide a corrective emotional experience in this way for those who may have been previously shamed for relapse. Providers can also support women in tolerating failure. They can offer support to increase coping, and work with the individual on accessing external resources such as social roles, housing, employment, and education. Therapists must be available and trustworthy in times of crisis, and provide a range of treatment options per the woman's choice. For example, one woman's plan might include her preferred medications and places to be hospitalized.

A Wellness Recovery Action Plan (WRAP) group may amplify the woman's personal coping, strengths, and mechanisms for staying well (Copeland, 1997). A WRAP group is normally peer-led and involves the development of recovery tools, advance directives, safety and crisis plans, and other resources. WRAP is also an evidence-based practice that has been evaluated and refined based on research outcomes (Jonikas et al., 2013). Some of the inherent value of WRAP is that the plan is developed and written by the woman and can then be shared with a provider, other team members, or natural supports.

Offering interventions in a noncoercive or nonpunitive way can be incredibly meaningful to women engaged in the recovery process. Many people in recovery typically experience some challenges with receiving evidence-based practice due to the lack of access to this specialized care. It is important to either provide these resources or offer referrals (Corrigan, Steiner, McCracken, Blaser, & Barr, 2001). Diverse interventions include but are not limited to the following:

- dialectical behavior therapy
- mindfulness-based stress reduction
- behavioral family therapy, peer specialists
- cognitive-behavioral therapy
- metacognitive therapy
- social skills training
- cognitive restructuring for trauma
- open dialogue approach
- supported employment
- supportive housing
- psychosocial interventions for alcohol and substance use disorders
- psychosocial interventions for weight management
- assertive community treatment
- psychodynamic psychotherapy.

Empirical evidence has found that these interventions, among others, are likely to help individuals in their wellness journey (Bellack, Mueser, Gingerich, & Agresta, 2013; Bergstrom et al., 2018; de Jong et al., 2019; Dixon et al., 2009; Dutton, Bermudez, Matas, Majid, & Myers, 2013; Johnson, et al., 2018; Kreyenbuhl, Buchanan, Dickerson, & Dixon, 2010; Lecomte, 2018; Linehan, 2014; Mueser & Glynn, 1995; Mueser et al., 2018; Rosenbaum, Alberdi, Haahr, Lindhardt, & Urferparnas, 2019). It is crucial to provide and offer these resources in ways that are not coercive. A forced approach is not likely to have positive outcomes and may further marginalize or retraumatize an individual.

Women in recovery can be encouraged to develop a positive sense of identity (Slade, 2009). Providers can help women make sense of their experience of what mental illness means to them as a person, without making assumptions about how they may see it. This offers the woman in recovery the psychological space to put this experience in context in her own life, develop personal responsibility, and build tools for coping. There are a number of messages that can be harmful, such as the idea that her life will be a certain, negative way; that mental illness means she is flawed; that she will not be able to pursue her dreams. However, with a hope-inspiring, nonjudgmental approach, much is possible.

It is important to engage women in conversations about how they uniquely experience the symptoms of their mental illness and any fluctuations related to their menstrual cycle. Women experience hormonal changes and concerns during breastfeeding or pregnancy. Prescribing should involve a careful assessment of the experiences of the individual woman in the context of her medication regimen, balanced with what the scientific literature recommends. Providers of psychotherapy and other team members such as peer specialists can amplify the woman's voice as they conceptualize how best to communicate her needs to a prescriber. A holistic approach is recommended, including assessing the woman's physical well-being and longevity (Brown et al., 1999; Chang et al., 2011). Holistic care includes support for a healthy diet, attending to substance use, smoking reduction, and implementing exercise. It is also vital to monitor challenges that may develop from medication effects such as metabolic syndrome, weight gain, increased prolactin levels, suicidality, akathisia, and other related concerns (Druss et al., 2018). Providers may also find it helpful to utilize the clinical worksheet located at the end of the chapter, "My Recovery Journey," with women with SMI and others who may benefit.

CONCLUSION

A recovery-oriented perspective recognizes the value of developing meaning and supporting autonomy. Providers must take into consideration the unique biological differences among women with SMI and how they experience illness, wellness, and particular life experiences such as pregnancy and hormonal changes in order to provide recovery-oriented and gender-sensitive services. This recovery orientation will allow optimal clinical engagement and best serve women with SMI.

CLINICAL STRATEGIES

- Assess the woman's experience of mental illness and make a supportive, therapeutic alliance that allows for processing of positive identity development.
- Avoid negative messages that the woman's life is flawed due to her mental illness or that she cannot pursue her dreams. Rather, affirm her strengths and hold hope for her as she works through difficult experiences and strives to develop a life of meaning.
- Assess from a person-centered perspective what goals in life carry personal meaning and make these the center of direction for the therapeutic process. This includes taking medications, going to therapy appointments, or going to groups. Focus on supporting women in pursuing personally meaningful activities (e.g., earning a college degree, finding a partner, becoming a chef, learning to skateboard, or taking up knitting).
- In therapy, set the agenda together. This empowers a woman to feel that she is in the "driver's seat" of what happens in therapy.
- Aim to support the woman in setting holistic goals that include physical wellness and spiritual wellness, in addition to traditional mental health goals. Doing this can help her advocate for herself with prescribers, team members, and natural supports.
- Conduct role plays and assertiveness training as needed to inspire the woman to pursue her goals and embrace her personal agency.
- Provide evidence-based practices, including interventions and resources, that will improve coping, wellness, identity development, hope, quality of life, and meaning. If specific interventions are not offered at your site, be creative about a referral process that can provide such service connection.
- Provide education about the fluctuating symptoms of mental illness and how woman may experience the effects and the effectiveness of any prescribed medications.
- Encourage the use of shared decision-making models on inter-professional and interdisciplinary teams.
- Avoid coercive or punitive forms of treatment, which may further disenfranchise a woman in recovery.
- Understand the therapy experience as more than a "fifty-minute hour" of talk therapy, but one that includes social justice practices of advocacy for the rights, legal support, housing, employment, and safety supports of a woman in recovery.
- Support the woman in recovery in developing and enhancing natural supports that provide fulfilling connection.

DISCUSSION QUESTIONS

1. What are the different mechanisms in therapy that can help transfer the concept of hope to a woman in recovery when she feels hopeless? How does this differ based on varying social locations such as the woman's socioeconomic status, intellectual level, employment history, housing status, and educational attainment?

2. How does one advocate for the provision of recovery-oriented care in a system that communicates negative messages to people with mental health problems, focusing on their symptoms, limitations, and poor prognoses? What resources or partners would be helpful to include in this process? What barriers to recovery-oriented care occur within the traditional mental health system?

3. What responsibility do you believe systems of care have in balancing psychotropic prescribing with the risk of health effects from medications? What tools do you think might be most helpful in considering the preferences, experiences, and goals of a woman in recovery as she thinks about communicating her views on taking medications with her team and/or prescriber?

4. What increased assessment experiences can systems of care develop so that they pay attention to the unique needs of every woman that they accept into treatment?

ACTIVITIES

Break into two groups and discuss the following topics for fifteen minutes. Then share as an entire group. Assign a scribe to take notes and a reporter to share takeaway points from the discussion. As the two groups reconvene, discuss any differences or similarities that came up as a group and expand on those ideas.

1. How do you switch the therapeutic alignment with a treatment team on an inpatient unit that has been engaging with a patient from a pathologizing or "this is what is wrong with you" approach to a recovery-oriented approach? Consider how that shift may occur when working with these women:
   - A woman who, ten years ago, killed her mother when she thought her mother was an alien but has not been violent since
   - A woman from a well-off family who has been abandoned by the family and is now on public assistance
   - A woman who has a history of trauma and starts to yell, between 9 and 11 every night, that someone is coming to beat her
   - A woman who likes to garden and frequently waters the plants at the hospital, so that the janitor can't keep track of how much water the plants are getting.

2. During the process of recovery, individuals seek to enhance their autonomy, personal agency, and sense of control, which are vital to assuming responsibility and directing their recovery journey. How do you envision mental health systems getting in the way of this at times, and how can this be navigated in pursuit of a more recovery-consistent orientation? Consider different elements such as:
   - Policies related to smoking
   - How medications are prescribed
   - Treatment engagement requisites (e.g., requirement to participate in groups, token economies)
   - Choices in hospitalization.

3. Though systems of mental health care have improved in their ability to offer more trauma-informed care, there are still many procedures in the mental health system that are experienced as aversive or traumatic. What are your ideas for helping shape the field in relation to the use of the following:
   - Seclusion/restraint
   - Level systems on an inpatient unit to gain privileges
   - Privacy in hospital settings
   - How treatment teams discuss patient information and how rounds are carried out

My Recovery Journey Worksheet

Domains in the Recovery Process	Needs and Strengths
Do I have hope?	
Do I have a voice in this process?	
How do I cope when I don't feel well?	
What people do I feel supported by?	
What do I need my providers to know?	
Do I know who I am?	
What are my strengths and skills?	
What activities do I have in my life that I love?	
What makes a life meaningful to me?	
How do I think about exercise in the context of my recovery?	
What structure do I need or is helpful to me?	
What are my concerns related to the physical effects of my medication?	
What is the next step in my journey?	

4

Motherhood, Family, and Relationships for Women with Serious Mental Illness

Our relationships with others are among the most important aspects of life. Interpersonal relationships have been found to be especially valuable for individuals in recovery (Spaniol et al., 2002). Increased social connectedness is associated with positive recovery outcomes (Spaniol et al., 2002; Tew et al., 2012). However, people with serious mental illness (SMI) frequently have fewer meaningful relationships (Macdonald et al., 2005). Furthermore, the literature indicates that some of these social interactions are not experienced as positive and can actually hinder the recovery process (Mezzina et al., 2006; Tew et al., 2006; Yanos et al., 2001). The chronic social rejection faced by women with mental illness can have devastating consequences.

Specifically, demeaning social interactions can lead people with SMI to withdraw from society (Topor et al., 2006). This is not surprising given the stigma and marginalization that those with SMI can face. Therefore, it is of particular importance to pay attention to the relational experiences of those with SMI and to foster healthy interactions that are conducive to recovery. Women with SMI may deal with a range of challenges in their relationships, such as motherhood, friendship, family, and dating. Though these relationships are of great value, the complexity of navigating these dynamics is not frequently explored in the literature on women with SMI (Padgett, Henwood, Abrams, & Drake, 2008).

For many individuals in recovery, it is difficult to achieve and maintain social connectedness due to a variety of factors, such as fear of others, isolation, underdeveloped social skills, and odd behavior. Or other intersecting experiences could interfere with social integration, such as a lack of social currency due to homelessness, trauma, living in disadvantaged neighborhoods, legal involvement, and lack of employment (Davidson et al., 2001; Morgan, Burns, Fitzpatrick, Pinfold, & Priebe, 2007; Padgett et al., 2008; Phelan & Link, 2004; Scheff, 1966; Ware et al., 2007). The literature also indicates that for people with schizophrenia, more severe negative symptoms are linked to smaller social networks (Goldberg, Rollins, & Lehman, 2003).

A qualitative study of 41 individuals dually diagnosed with SMI and substance use disorders shed light on relationship experiences among this group (Padgett et al., 2008). The researchers identified themes of isolation, family conflict, barriers to pursuing a domestic partner, and a challenge to find positive relationships. Many people identified themselves as loners who did not get close to people. Some of this distancing occurred because of losses experienced in the past and/or a lack of ability to trust others. Other individuals reported greater social isolation and withdrawal from social relationships as symptoms flared up, such as mania or depression. The participants also isolated at times out of a need for greater privacy. Despite this need, they continued to seek relationships, but on their own terms. Interestingly, the researchers did not find a link between stronger social connectedness and positive outcomes. This finding points to the necessity of understanding the type and nature of social connectedness that is conducive to recovery. The participants reported that familial relationships had to be constantly negotiated and came with ups and downs. This confirms the data on close relationships, where overly intrusive, critical, or hostile family behavior is actually associated with relapse for individuals with SMI (Hooley, 2007).

The participants in the qualitative study by Padgett and colleagues (2008) predominantly described that other goals came before a domestic partner. However, there was a common desire for romantic relationships, though many wanted to get their lives together first or felt other things had to be taken care of before that experience could occur. Despite the need and desire to make positive relational connections, this is difficult for those with SMI given their lack of capacity to move out of areas where they are surrounded by the distractions of drug use, poverty, crime, and others in desperate need as well. These social issues clarify other findings that suggest that social distancing may sometimes facilitate recovery as well (Sells, Stayner, & Davidson, 2004).

WOMEN WITH SMI AND RELATIONSHIPS

Though the literature indicates that relationships with others help develop the self-esteem and development of women, many women with SMI report a lack of those relationships (Chernomas, Clarke, & Chisholm, 2000; Miller & Stiver, 1997). In one study of gender differences of individuals with SMI, women reported personal relationships as more formative and important to them than men did, and women put more emphasis on these relationships (Ritsher, Coursey, & Farrell, 1997). In that study, these relationships were more important to the women than even their experience and journey with SMI itself. In fact, many women have shared that connecting with others specifically after having been given a diagnosis of an SMI was incredibly meaningful. In a related study, women with schizophrenia discussed the value of relationships and their challenges with connecting with others in meaningful ways (Chernomas et al., 2000). These women also found that making new friends or reestablishing prior connections can be daunting and emotionally threatening.

Women with SMI also contend with different relational demands and expectations from their diverse relationships such as those within a mothering relationship, friendships, family, and intimate partnerships (Ackerson, 2003; Gove, 1984; Sands, 1995). Women have higher sociocultural expectations in comparison to men in terms of caregiving roles (Gove, 1984). Women with SMI are twice as likely as their male counterparts to be a parent (Nicholson, Nason, Calabresi, & Yando, 1999). They are also more likely to be in a caregiving role, such as with a sick family member, which is a role that involves psychological distress and demands (Gove, 1984).

Motherhood

Women with SMI have varying experiences with motherhood. Some women find an inherent value in the mothering relationship, which gives purpose to their lives (Nicholson & Biebel, 2002). Many of these women deal with particular risks to their mood during pregnancy and after (Park, Solomon, & Mandell, 2006). Others, however, may encounter significant difficulties in motherhood, such as guilt about not being able to care for their children and loss of custody (Montgomery, Tompkins, Forchuk, & French, 2006; Oyserman, Mowbray, Meares, & Firminger, 2000).

Women with SMI also tend to have health factors that have to be navigated in their pregnancies (Mowbray, Oyserman, Zemencuk, & Ross, 1995). The literature indicates that a major barrier to safer sex practices and contraceptive use among individuals with mental illness is a lack of knowledge (Cook, 2000). A review of medical records of 56 women discharged from a psychiatric ward showed a dearth of information provided to them on sexual health or contraception (Cole, 2000). Higher rates of miscarriage have also been reported among women with SMI, and there are serious concerns about continuing to take psychotropic medication during pregnancy (Mowbray et al., 1995). Women with psychiatric histories are also more likely to experience postpartum psychiatric issues compared to those with no prior history.

Mothers with SMI are less likely to receive good prenatal care, are more likely to have difficulties with drug and alcohol use, and are more likely to have difficulties fulfilling the basic needs of their children on an everyday basis (Park et al., 2006). Many have difficulties dealing with stress and discipline. They often report a lack of satisfaction with the parenting relationship, yet regularly seek support due to a fear of losing custody. Though women with SMI are more likely to lose custody of their children compared to their female counterparts, the evidence suggests that they are not more prone to abuse their children (Miller & Finnerty, 1996). In one study of 322 women with SMI, 26% of the women lost custody of their children at some point. In another study, 48% of women with SMI had children in foster care compared to only 2% in a control group (Miller & Finnerty, 1996; Sands,

Koppelman, & Solomon, 2004). Ironically, the mothers with SMI who had contact with and support from psychiatric care were more likely to have had a loss of custody (Park et al., 2006). Many of these women likely had opportunities to receive support for their parenting needs. However, this is quite rare, and it is no wonder some women are reticent to seek treatment if they have children (Diaz-Caneja & Johnson, 2004; Park et al., 2006). The consequences are grave, if reaching out for help could lead to the potential loss of custody of your children.

Overall, women with SMI in the Miller and Finnerty (1996) study were more than four times as likely to have lost custody of their children than women without a mental illness. Additionally, African American women were more likely than White American women to have involvement with child welfare services, but not more likely to have out-of-home placement. This evidence suggests the need for better coordination of care between mental health systems and the child welfare system. These findings also suggest that many women with SMI may not understand their parenting rights and need support to navigate these experiences (Park et al., 2006; Sands et al., 2004).

Though many women with SMI desire to become mothers, a number of providers in the mental health field have historically held a pathological view toward this desire that needs to be remedied (Nicholson & Beibel, 2002). Though some view women with SMI as incompetent to fulfill this role, other literature indicates that with the help of innovative services, this role can be successfully attained and maintained (Nicholson & Biebel, 2002; Walsh, MacMillan, & Jamieson, 2002).

A qualitative study indicates that women engage in many efforts to have close relationships with their children despite their challenges with illness (Montgomery et al., 2006). Furthermore, mothers reported choosing strategies to hide the illness or mask it to protect their children and their parenting roles. Women were also likely to try to portray an ideal image as mothers despite the serious challenges they were experiencing. One can imagine how important this perception is to many women given the real risk they face of losing custody of their children. Themes that emerged related to trying to appear normal, creating security, and being responsible. The women found these strategies to keep their children were important but exhausting.

To address the need for more research on mothers with SMI, one of these authors (Mizock) conducted a qualitative study to explore the experiences of mothers with SMI as well as women with SMI who did not become parents (Mizock, Merg, Boyle, & Kompaniez-Dunigan, in press; Table 4.1). The following themes emerged:

Motherhood Declined: intentional decision not to have children
Motherhood Derailed: disruption in plans to have children
Motherhood Disabled: unable to have children
Motherhood Reimagined: parenting role was adapted to accommodate
     motherhood

Table 4.1 QUALITATIVE THEMES PERTAINING TO PARENTING/MOTHERHOOD
EXPERIENCES OF WOMEN WITH SMI ($N = 20$)

Themes	Definitions
Motherhood Declined	Decision to become intentionally childless among women with SMI.
Motherhood Derailed	Disruption of plans to become a mother among women with SMI.
Motherhood Disabled	Incapacitation of ability to be a mother among women with SMI.
Motherhood Reimagined	Adaptations to parenting role to accommodate mothering in the face of obstacles among women with SMI.
Mattering through Motherhood	Self-preservation and meaning found in mothering among women with SMI.

From Mizock et al. (in press). Reprinted with permission from *Psychiatric Rehabilitation Journal* © 2019.

Mattering Through Motherhood: ways women found meaning and sought survival through parenting.

The study findings suggested that women with SMI face several specific challenges with respect to parenting. Some may opt out of parenting as a way to nurture themselves and potential unborn children. Others may find self-preservation by protecting their children from domestic violence and the violence directed at one-self in the form of suicide.

Some women with SMI describe motherhood as a unifying force that keeps them devoted to treatment. They find motherhood brings them a sense of purpose and dedication to engagement in their recovery journey. Similarly, many women with SMI report that being a mother is an outlet for emotional expression and is also a valued social role (Mowbray, Oyserman, & Ross, 1995; Oyserman, Bybee, Mowbray, & Khang, 2000; Perkins, 1992). In this respect, the parent identity provides a purpose and anchor for many women and helps push them forward in their recovery.

Though some studies indicate women with SMI are, now more than ever, carrying out parenting and mothering responsibilities, they are also frequently dealing with problems associated with single parenting, poverty, and poor living arrangements, as well as child behavior problems (Mowbray, Oyserman, Bybee, MacFarlane, & Rueda-Riedle, 2001). Despite these challenges, women with SMI still describe motherhood as a key source of fulfillment in their lives. However, most psychiatric facilities do not address these interests, and less than one-third of mental health authorities note the status of the children of their patients in their records. When asked about the changes that have occurred in their lives due to motherhood, many women reported a sense of personal worth and accomplishment, positive behavioral consequences such as ending destructive relationships or ending drug use, and a positive impact in managing their mental illness, with some enhancement in social status and role (Mowbray et al., 2001). In this same study, only 10% of mothers gave more negative responses such as worries about children, financial problems, and a loss of freedom.

Many women may fear passing a mental illness onto an unborn child, or being unable to care for a child due to mental illness, which may lead some women to choose not to become a mother (Anderson, 2014; Mizock et al., 2019). For some, it may be a relief not to procreate and not to experience the burden or associated anxiety or fear that may come along with the responsibility of parenting, while navigating their recovery journey. Other research indicates that current stresses, functioning, and social support, rather than diagnosis, has the most impact on positive parenting attitudes and behavior such as involvement with children's education and nurturance (Oyserman, Bybee, & Mowbray, 2000).

Friendship

Not surprisingly, friendships are also an important source of connection for women with SMI (Chernomas et al., 2000; Spaniol et al., 2002). In a study among individuals with SMI, women were more likely than men to say they had a best friend (70% vs. 44%), and a greater percentage of women reported a mutually equitable relationship with another individual (72% vs. 58%) (Ritsher et al., 1997). This may reflect feminist research about how women and men are socialized differently per relational theory. Relational theory posits that when women experience more positive, mutual relationships, they will have more self-worth (Miller, 2008).

One study shows that better social support decreases the length of time it takes for psychiatric symptoms to remit in women with major depression (Kendler, Walters, & Kessler, 1997). Other studies indicate that this is correlated with a positive recovery process (Tew et al., 2012). However, it may help to clarify the nuances of these types of relational experiences for women with SMI. Studies show that people with SMI can face problems with their current friendships and/ or redeveloping old friendships after receiving a diagnosis (Chernomas et al., 2000). For example, it is crucial to the recovery process to have choice in these type of relationships and friendships. Ties that are supportive and meaningful are most important, versus ones that may be more critical or induce experiences of stigma (Hendryx, Green, & Perrin, 2009; Tew et al., 2006; Yanos et al., 2006).

Multiple research studies show that social network size and social support are correlated with a better sense of recovery for those with SMI (Corrigan & Phelan, 2004; Hendryx et al., 2009; Pevalin & Goldberg, 2003). Benefits include emotional, psychological, and material gains, including motivational encouragement and modeling (Breier & Strauss, 1984). More recent research shows that a greater range of activities with others may lead to a better reported experience of recovery, especially when social support was lower before study engagement (Hendryx et al., 2009). Furthermore, these social experiences can occur under a range of circumstances, from inside or outside the home, for more or less socially and physically active individuals. In fact, the empirical evidence highlights how having a choice and an individualized nature to the support may be one of the most important aspects of developing relationships and building a sense of control over one's life. This literature points to the importance of social network, size, and choice in friendships for women with SMI.

Many people with SMI experience most of their interpersonal contact in their mental health services (Wong, Matejkowski, & Lee, 2011). However, researchers suggest that these social relationships within mental health services are not experienced as having the important quality of reciprocity. These settings are not ones in which consumers have been able to engage in mutually reciprocal roles, given the formal nature of the way services are provided and the way they are not commensurate (Wong et al., 2011). This gives insight into the need for more opportunities for people with SMI to develop mutually supportive relationships. Experiencing mutuality in relationships also provides opportunities for women to not only exercise choice, but to give back to others. This may be particularly valuable as some women with SMI may be unable to fulfill some of the traditional caregiving roles they are expected to perform.

Family Relationships and Dynamics

The researchers of the well-known Schizophrenia Patient Outcomes Research Team recommend family support and psychoeducation as among the most important treatments for individuals with SMI (Kreyenbuhl, Buchanan, Dickerson, & Dixon, 2009). Many people with SMI receive their primary support and care through their family (Kohn-Wood & Wilson, 2005; Wynaden et al., 2006). Many individuals also experience complexities in these familial relationships as they may be burdened with over-intrusiveness, negative emotionality, and hostility, all of which are components of high expressed emotion, which can have negative effects on people with SMI (Scazufca & Kuipers, 1998). This association may be linked to challenges people have with processing complex emotions and sustaining attention in emotionally charged situations, but the science does indicate a correlation with relapse and rehospitalization (Dixon, Adams, & Lucksted, 2000; Scazufca & Kuipers, 1998).

Many women with SMI may feel pressure to accept traditional family roles such as caring for an ill or elderly family member, which can add stress (Mizock, Salmonsen, & Smith, under review). There also may be pressure from family members to conduct unpaid work inside the home and take care of children or other family members if they cannot work outside the home. Interestingly, more men than women with SMI reported having at least one family member who was supportive to them (64% vs. 55%), and more men than women reported feeling like a fully accepted member of their family (72% vs. 61%) (Ritsher et al., 1997). These findings may be explained by the extra societal expectations and burdens put on women at home. Many women with SMI may feel more familial burdens and less acceptance of their illness or divergence from serving in traditional familial roles.

The evidence suggests that families of a person with SMI that use more problem-solving strategies and coping behaviors work better as a family unit and are less problematic for the individual with SMI (Saunders, 1999). Strategies such as seeking spiritual support, reframing experiences, mobilizing resources, being aware of internal and external patterns, and developing social support have been shown to be elements of well-functioning families of people with SMI.

There is some interesting research among individuals with SMI that indicates that the amount of support patients give parents and siblings is associated with the level of support they receive back. In essence, providing support to other family members is the strongest predictor of the level of family support in return (Horwitz, Reinhard, & Howell-White, 1996). This study indicates that it may be worthwhile to examine caregiving in families of those with SMI as a process of mutual exchange, which would also support the value reported by those with SMI themselves of being in mutually reciprocal relationships (Wong et al., 2011). However, this would have to be contextualized on an individual basis given that this mutuality would best be a choice for the individual with SMI and would have positive relational benefits or it could pose added psychological and physical burdens. This may be especially true given that many women report that they feel undue stress and pressure to be caregivers and providers of intense support to other family members, which may not always be conducive to their recovery process.

Based on empirical evidence, those with SMI provide their family with significant contributions, such as offering companionship, doing household chores, shopping, providing news about family members, and listening to problems (Greenberg, Greenley, & Benedict, 1994). It is important to acknowledge the roles that individuals with SMI play in their families.

Dating

The experience of SMI may interfere with finding a partner and feelings of relational self-efficacy. Though in most Western adult cultures having a romantic relationship is a normative developmental trajectory, individuals with SMI persistently have challenges with developing and maintaining intimate partner relationships (Carey et al., 2001; Wright, Wright, Perry, & Foote-Ardah, 2007). Frequently, the relationships of those with SMI are short or episodic (Dickerson et al., 2004). Many people may have difficulty finding a partner due to the cultural stigma of mental illness and the societal belief that those with SMI are dangerous and socially unpredictable (Phelan et al., 2000). Researchers have found that expectations of rejection and discrimination may produce feelings of being tentative and ineffective in social interactions, contributing to negative evaluation by others (Farina et al., 1968; Farina et al., 1971; Link, 1987).

Other theories about the challenges that people have related to developing a romantic relationship may be linked to a reduction in libido due to symptoms, while others argue it is the medications that reduce sexual functioning (Wright et al., 2007). Many clinicians also view their clients as asexual or consider sexual relationships to be inappropriate for them; such providers may believe that people in recovery cannot maintain a positive partnership and project the ideology that sexual behavior is another challenge to be treated (Buckley et al., 1999; Hogan, 1980; Pinderhughes, Barrabee, & Reyna, 1972).

It is also relevant to note that women with SMI are at an increased risk for intimate partner violence (Cascardi, Mueser, DeGiralomo, & Murrin, 1996; Dickerson et al., 2004). Many women with SMI experience coercive sexual engagements and become caught up in sex exchange (Meade & Sikkema, 2005). Because they hold less sociopolitical power, many women with SMI are likely to encounter barriers to developing and maintaining a healthy intimate partner relationship. These risks may carry negative consequences for women with SMI. For example, in an empirical study of women with SMI, a correlation was found with stigma and several correlates of HIV risk, such as exchanging sex for money or material items, having more than one sexual partner, and using substances before sex (Collins, Sweetland, & Zybert, 2007).

Many participants in a qualitative study reported that they had lost relationships with romantic partners due to their mental illness and experience sexual discrimination (Wright et al., 2007). Many women in this study reported feeling like they have little choice in relationships and have a fear of "coming out" about their mental illness with prospective partners, feeling undersired or devalued, leading to anticipated stigma. Relatedly, according to the literature, stigma also impacts the choice of dating or sexual partners by women (Davison & Huntington, 2010). In this respect, women with SMI may be prone to choose partners with similar mental health experiences or partners that will be accepting of their experiences. Women also report having challenges with sexual functioning due to symptoms and to medication side effects, causing great disruption with relationships, including challenges with libido and inorgasmia (Cook, 2000; Sullivan, 1993). Women with schizophrenia may have less long-lasting sexual relationships due to the impact of antipsychotics on sexual functioning. A recent review shows that risperidone and classical antipsychotics are associated with higher frequencies of sexual dysfunction; clozapine, olanzapine, quetiapine, and aripiprazole have a lesser impact (de Boer, Castelein, Wiersma, Schoevers, & Knegtering, 2015). Strategies to deal with sexual dysfunction might include psychoeducation, relationship counseling, and/or pharmacologic strategies such as lowering the dosage, switching to a prolactin-sparing antipsychotic, or adding a dopamine agonist. However, these issues do not appear to be routinely addressed by prescribers.

To address this gap in the research, one of these authors (Mizock) conducted a qualitative study (Mizock, DeMartini, LaMar, & Stringer, 2019) to investigate the dating experiences of women with SMI. Several themes were identified (Table 4.2):

Table 4.2 QUALITATIVE THEMES PERTAINING TO WORK EXPERIENCES OF WOMEN
WITH SMI (*N* = 20)

Themes	Definitions
Function Matching	The challenge women with SMI may face in finding a partner at a similar level of mental health functioning.
Pathologizing Problems	The tendency of some partners of women with SMI to dismiss their complaints about the relationship and attribute their negative emotions to their mental illness.
Symptom Interference	Instances in which the mental health symptoms of a woman with SMI could interfere with the development and maintenance of a relationship.
Dating Deal Breakers	Dating barriers due to stigma for women with SMI, either through internalized stigma blocking the pursuit of dating, or external stigma leading to rejection.
Sexual Foreclosure	An obstacle in the romantic relationships of women with SMI as a result of giving up on sexual intimacy, often as a result of trauma, mental health symptoms, or side effects of psychiatric medication.
Dating Deprioritized	The phenomenon of women with SMI to reduce the importance of dating in their lives, or forgo it altogether.

From Mizock et al. (2019). Reprinted with permission from *Journal of Relationships Research* © 2019.

Function Matching: Women with SMI may face challenges in finding a partner at a similar level of mental health functioning.

Pathologizing Problems: Some partners of women with SMI tend to dismiss their complaints about the relationship and attribute their negative emotions to the mental illness.

Symptom Interference: Mental health symptoms of a woman with SMI could intrude on the development and maintenance of a relationship.

Dating Deal Breakers: Dating barriers occurred due to stigma, either through internalized stigma blocking the pursuit of dating or external stigma leading to rejection.

Sexual Foreclosure: Women with SMI may give up on sexual intimacy, often as a result of trauma, mental health symptoms, or side effects of psychiatric medication.

Dating Deprioritized: Women with SMI may reduce the importance of dating in their lives, or forgo it altogether.

Overall, the study found that stigma and mental health symptoms had considerable impact on the romantic and intimate relationships of women with SMI. Women with SMI demonstrated a range of decision-making and relational strategies to enhance recovery and resilience in their life. At times, these strategies helped them to pursue and prioritize their relationship goals, while at other times these women appeared to decide to forgo dating altogether.

Deegan (2001) has advocated that individuals with SMI have the need and desire for intimacy, love, and companionship just like the rest of humanity, and therefore these concerns and goals should be taken more seriously in our communities and systems of care. Such important relationships are seen as a vital part of the recovery journey of many people; therefore, it is a social justice issue to support these goals for women with SMI. Providing positive and safe mechanisms for meeting others and engaging in dating may help women in recovery with this process. Dating and intimate partner relationships could produce benefits of mutual caring and support that should not be overlooked.

COMPLEXITY OF RELATIONAL DYNAMICS

Women with SMI face a complex constellation of experiences as they move forward on their recovery journey and navigate their relational goals. They may experience stigma and rejection that they have not experienced before they dealt with a diagnosis of mental illness. Therefore, they may have to navigate those dynamics and deal with feelings about mistreatment. At worst, this can lead to the internalization of such rejection. At best, these experiences offer women empowerment as they make personal choices about what relationships they want in their life or do not. In this next section, some case narratives will provide a picture of how women with SMI may experience different complexities in their interpersonal relationships.

CASE NARRATIVES

Case 1: Kya

"Kya" is a 21-year-old Ghanaian woman who came to the United States with her family when she was eight years old. She completed high school and graduated with honors. She enrolled in college, declaring a major in biochemistry with a plan to go to medical school. She finished three years of school and was doing well until she started to hear unusual voices that told her to go to the top of her apartment building and stand on the ledge looking over the city. She listened to the voices on several occasions and went to the top of her apartment building, contemplating walking on the ledge. While she did not jump off, it was a frightening experience. Her family helped her seek an intake at a local mental health agency and she started engaging in treatment there.

Thankfully, the mental health agency had a first-episode clinic that was well versed in working with young adults experiencing some of the first signs of psychosis. She started working in outpatient psychotherapy with a therapist well trained in working with people with first-episode psychosis. Her psychiatrist was part of an interdisciplinary team that worked collaboratively with her. The clinic also had a strong focus on family therapy, but there were many difficulties that arose for Kya in this area. Her family wanted her to move home immediately so they could look after her and provide her with adequate support. They also felt concerned that she could not continue with classes and that the stress of school might be too much for her to deal with.

However, Kya wanted to continue her classes. She had begun psychotherapy and was taking medication to help manage her voices. Kya felt distressed that her family was already starting to see her differently from the way they used to (as their star student and part of their future). She wanted to pursue her hopes and dreams and saw her experience as just part of her life journey. Kya also was concerned that her family might think she would be unable to make it to medical school, and she did not want to let them down. She was worried that this was possible if she had more troubling episodes in the future. Kya wanted to reassure them that she could still work toward her goals and dreams despite these challenges, but she also wanted to ask for more psychological space to think through the type of support she needed from them. She didn't feel she could be completely honest with most of her friends about her experience with psychosis, as she felt many of them might be rude or hurtful and think of her as "crazy." Kya found herself pulling away from most of her peer relationships, aside from one of her closest friends whom she felt could support her through this experience.

Kya found one of the most difficult aspects of her mental health challenges to be diagnostic stigma. She explored the issue of stigma with her therapist. The therapist helped her identify what she felt she needed most from her relationships in order to continue with the dreams she had for her life. This meant putting parameters around her family's plans to pull her out of school. Instead, Kya asked her family to serve in a supportive role in her pursuit of her goals rather than making decisions for her. Her family respected her wishes.

The first-episode clinic was able to use person-centered treatment planning (Tondora, Miller, Slade, & Davidson, 2014) to work with Kya's family and providers to discuss and plan how best to support her. Kya was also connected to the re-sources of a peer-run decision support center, which helps people in recovery to take the lead in their decision-making process (Deegan, Rapp, Holter, & Reifer, 2008). These approaches helped her voice her needs and preferences regarding con-tinuing in her studies. These supports also helped her to explore the medications that could best support her goal of maintaining her cognitive capacity while aiding her in managing distressing voices. These supports also helped different members of her treatment team and family know what roles to serve in this process.

Case 2: Emmie

"Emmie" is a 50-year-old Asian American woman who has struggled with severe depression and suicidality throughout her life. These problems worsened after she gave birth to her two children. Emmie dealt with depression throughout high school. She also had one suicide attempt at age 18 after losing her best friend in a car accident. Her family had a difficult time talking about the attempt openly, but did help her to seek mental health services afterward. At that time, she began seeing a regular therapist and taking psychiatric medication. Emmie became quite angry at times and felt that it took her trying to commit suicide for her family to help her get care, even though she had told them many times that she felt depressed. This built some resentment in Emmie and also fear that now they would monitor her too much or not trust her because of the suicide attempt. Emmie went on to college and engaged in student health services at her own initiation, which helped her to address her depression and suicidal ideation. She earned a degree in chemistry, then a Ph.D., and had an excellent teaching job at a university.

Emmie married in her early 30s and had two children. After the birth of her children she developed more problems with depression and suicidal ideation. She was hospitalized multiple times and took a few years off from work. She also had two suicide attempts while the children were little. Her husband and family took care of the children while she was in the hospital and over the next few years. Throughout this time, Emmie grew to feel that her parents were making parenting decisions regarding her children without her.

Over many years, Emmie came to spend less time in the hospital and more time engaging in work and her personal goals, including taking care of her children at home while the children were in primary school and high school. However, Emmie voiced struggles with her family at different times in navigating the expectations and differentiation of roles, given her experiences with depression and suicidality. She felt they were too infantilizing and took away from her role as mother. At other times, when they expected her to be doing well, she felt they did not help in ways they could so she did not become overwhelmed with childrearing and could focus on her work and recovery. Emmie worried that her children looked to their grandmother and father more for guidance and boundaries than they did to her. She found her feelings to be in conflict with her culture's tradition to follow the decisions made by her elders. Ultimately, Emmie wanted to increase her rights to make decisions regarding her household, even though she had faced some serious wellness challenges, and this differed from her cultural background.

As Emmie's children went off to college, the dynamic shifted to the adult children talking predominantly on the phone to her husband and mother about any problems or challenges at school. She felt they tiptoed around her. Emmie became quite frustrated and worked on these dynamics within the context of her individual psychotherapy. Her therapist had worked with Emmie for the prior 10 years and had helped her to communicate her needs and desires with her family. The therapist worked within the family's cultural dynamics as an Asian American family and helped Emmie to establish more differentiation. Emmie did not want her children to see her as fragile and wanted to be able to be a source of relational support. This meant acknowledging that she does suffer from depression and suicidal ideation but can tolerate her own affect regarding their problems as well.

Emmie's therapist integrated multicultural feminist therapy with behavioral family therapy. In this work, Emmie was able to set up structures that were supportive for her recovery as well with a therapy approach that was attentive to her family's culture (Worell & Remer, 2003). This was a complicated process and involved sharing some difficult emotional content. It was challenging to be open about some of these emotions as this was not something that was traditionally ascribed to. As the family members learned more about the needs of each another, they were able to support each other more effectively and with more reciprocity. Emmie came to find more satisfaction in these close relationships. This process did not occur overnight; the family worked toward such goals over 20 years as they grew accustomed to Emmie's needs.

Both Kya and Emmie's stories contain different perspectives and interpersonal dynamics that are important to understand. Kya experienced conflict with her family due to a difference in beliefs. She wanted to express her autonomous voice about her goals in life after experiencing her first episode of psychosis. Her family grew more open to this conversation and was able to respect her wishes, coming to agreement about their boundaries. Emmie's experience is complicated as she was dealing with multigenerational cultural dynamics with her parents, her own family, and her children. Emmie had to deal with depression and suicidality during the postpartum years and navigation of various sociocultural expectations of mothers. This was not something that was common for her family, and she had to work on the idea of therapy as a family unit. However, over time they were able to do this. This case highlights that relationships can wax and wane in their supportive and stressful nature, and this can be challenging for a woman in recovery. Therefore, providers should continually assess these dynamics throughout their clinical work to see what needs exist and what goals they should be working toward to facilitate the recovery process.

CLINICAL APPLICATIONS

Foundational Constructs

In this section, foundational components of relationships that appear to be conducive to recovery for women with SMI will be explored and clinical applications will be shared.

CHOICE
The fundamental element of choice in relationships seems to be one of the most important dynamics to consider for women with SMI. The literature supports the value of choice in relationships for people in recovery (Tew et al., 2006; Yanos et al., 2006). Women feel pressure from competing relational demands such as caring for children, ill family members, or older family members, expectations as a mother, and expectations as an intimate partner. Hence, it is important to deconstruct how to engage in choice. Some women struggle to meet typical

expectations of relationships, so it may be important to define their mutual expectations. This may be incredibly helpful for caretaking relationships such as with those who have traditional expectations for a mother. Some women may not be able to serve in those capacities at all due to being hospitalized or due to loss of custody. However, just because they may not physically be in the role of caring for their children's physical needs, it is vital not to overlook how a woman would like to proceed with her relationship with her child. For instance, what type of communication would she prefer (seeing them in person, visits, phone calls, letters, or email)? It is valuable to identify the parts of the parenting relationship she would like to fulfill and how to communicate the experiences she is going through so the child and other involved parties can become more understanding and supportive.

Having choice in how one engages with one's family of origin is essential. Women with SMI may experience a range of levels of support from their families. In some instances, family members may serve as conservators or payees for a woman with SMI. The woman may feel that she has lost her voice and must engage with those family members in the way that they demand. It is crucial to identify her preferences for engaging with her family, especially if she perceives a lack of choice. Women for whom conservators have been appointed may be particularly prone to silencing, and that is not the role of conservatorship (Probate Courts of Connecticut, 2008). In essence, conservators are supposed to help make specific decisions for individuals when they are unable to do so because of mental incapacity, but the decisions should still reflect the individuals' desires if their mental faculties were intact. Demands by family members for what the relationship should look like, such as visits, family therapy, or the woman in recovery should still inform family meetings. This is true for her goals for clinical services as well. Similarly, women should have a choice in how often, in what format, and in what manner they engage with family members. Sadly, this can be taken advantage of or ignored in many places of institutional care.

SAFETY

Relationship dynamics for women should include a sense of physical and psychological safety, given the likelihood of abuse. If a relationship does not feel safe and/or there has been abuse or violence in the relationship, it is helpful to conduct safety planning with the woman and the individual who enacts the violence so that this does not occur again. Safety planning should include connections to systems within which they interface, such as health care, criminal justice, shelter, or advocacy systems but also other community supports (Campbell, 2002, 2004). Systemic connection or the supporting mental health organization having a relationship with the prior perpetrator of violence and tracking growth shows better outcomes in the literature than not having contact with the perpetrator. Some research shows that women may be more likely to seek help from a family member or the police than from a health care provider or a domestic violence agency (Burke, Gielen, McDonnell, O'Campo, & Maman, 2001). It is important to support women in their recovery and process of developing safety in their relationships, as the literature indicates it is likely a process of recognizing that a relationship may be unsafe or abusive, setting boundaries, and/or ending a relationship.

Therefore, clinical work should not be conceptualized as supporting a woman during only one stage of this process, such as ending the relationship, as this may be a long process or may never occur. Making changes in these situations involves a complex psychological process that may take some time, but can also be built with safety strategies. The literature indicates that use of the transtheoretical stages of change model may be helpful to conceptualize this process of change. From this perspective, change may move from precontemplation (no recognition of problem), to contemplation (acknowledging a problem), to preparation (considering options), to action (selecting an option and taking action), and then maintenance (staying safe by using safety strategies) (Burke et al., 2001). It is also possible for a woman with SMI to move back and forth between stages as she thinks about change.

Support

Ideally, relationships should be supportive, and those that a woman in recovery does not feel are supportive should be examined. This can help increase insight and inform decisions about whether to continue that relationship and how that engagement should be constructed. A woman may feel the need to provide feedback and process her experience of a date, friendship, or family member with another individual and see if the relationship can grow and improve with appropriate feedback. If the relationship cannot improve, she should feel the freedom and support from others to do what is necessary to put boundaries around it or move on as she is able. This may be especially challenging when one may be involuntarily hospitalized or involuntarily medicated. In such cases, seeking out a patient advocate, peer support, appointed conservator, and legal representation may be useful. A number of interventions could be helpful toward achieving these goals, including the support of assertiveness training and empowerment models. Other interventions such as dialectical behavior therapy (DBT), which teaches interpersonal effectiveness and how to navigate such difficult dilemmas, may be helpful in these situations for women with SMI (Linehan, 2014).

Assessment

The research on interpersonal relationships for women with SMI suggests a number of related clinical implications. It is always valuable to assess and explore the relationships of women with SMI fully. For instance, though women might have many family members involved in their life, they may not all be supportive. In reality, some may be quite negative, intrusive, or even abusive. For other women with SMI, the most supportive relationships they have may be with a community member, a spiritual guide, or a friend. Those are the relationships they may want to deepen and depend on. They may also need support to establish boundaries with family members who are not supportive. A woman may need assistance from a mental health provider to identify her ideal characteristics in an intimate partner. She may need to develop safety strategies and enforce boundaries to avoid recurrence of intimate partner violence. Some women with SMI may realize that they are in an abusive relationship and would like information about how to work toward safety and/or trauma treatment.

Specific assessment tools that might be helpful from a recovery perspective include tools such as the Values in Action Inventory of Strengths (VIAS). The scale is housed within the Mental Health Statistics Improvement Program's Adult Consumer Satisfaction Survey (Peterson & Seligman, 2004; Shafer & Ang, 2018; Wilks, Heintz, & Lemieux, 2020). The VIAS is an online questionnaire that helps identify the respondent's signature strengths. It is non-illness-based and helps activate character traits that are useful and can also facilitate healthy relationships. The VIAS covers virtues such as courage, wisdom, humanity, justice, transcendence, and temperance.

The Perceived Social Connectedness scale has also been shown to be useful for individuals with schizophrenia and helps assess their social networks (Wilks et al., 2020). The recovery literature describes using the Appreciative Listening Cycle rather than a problem-focused cycle (Cooperrider & Whitney, 1999). From this perspective, an assessment of an individual involves the four steps of Discover, Dream, Design, and Destiny; these pertain to identifying passions, goals, and dreams; normalizing challenges related to attaining those goals; assessing resources; and facing challenges.

Psychosocial assessments of parenting status should explore the meaning the woman takes from parenting, which may be very different for each person (Mowbray et al., 2001; Oyserman et al., 2000). It is important to offer a safe space to evaluate this role for women with SMI as part of the recovery process.

Treatment Planning

Person-centered treatment planning is a good avenue for thinking about working toward the relational goals of a woman with SMI (Adams & Grieder, 2013). This is a service plan used to create a document for the clinical team that identifies the goals most important to the individual in recovery. It helps map out what the individual and the team need to do in order to move toward these goals. It includes amplifying supports chosen by the individual. Person-centered treatment planning should include specifics about navigating any concerns or goals a mother may have about parenting and the well-being of her children.

Therapeutic Strategies

There are many therapeutic strategies that can be useful to the relationship goals of women in recovery. Behavioral family therapy has a good evidence base and can help family members express emotions more appropriately, draw better boundaries, elevate the voice of the person in recovery, and develop better problem-solving and conflict-resolution skills (Mueser & Glynn, 1995). Lefley (2009) has reviewed model family psychoeducation interventions for people with SMI, finding strong empirical outcomes such as lower rehospitalization rates, better prognoses, and more well-being for family members.

Other therapies such as interpersonal process therapy and DBT may be useful to the relationship goals of women with SMI as well (Andrews, 2001; Linehan, 2014). Interpersonal process therapy may help a woman with SMI understand the interpersonal dynamics she experiences and can help her to see the therapeutic relationship as a microcosm of what she may experience interpersonally in the world. Therefore, the woman may be able to develop a greater understanding of her interpersonal functioning, develop more adaptive relational skills, experience corrective emotional experiences, and work toward her relational goals from the foundation of work within the therapeutic relationship.

DBT can also be helpful with the relationships of women with SMI, either in an individual therapy or in a skills group format. DBT can help increase assertiveness, become more effective in relationships, and manage emotions more effectively, while also working toward recovery goals (Linehan, 2014).

Psychotherapy integration (Stricker & Gold, 2013) and multicultural feminist therapy approaches can be integrated within the use of any of these therapeutic approaches. For example, one can integrate an egalitarian approach, understanding of the sociopolitical impact of challenges, cultural awareness and recognition of the intersectionality of experiences of the individual, and opportunities for empowerment (Enns, 2004). In addition, pathology can be reframed as not residing solely within the individual but as a problem with the sociopolitical context (Enns, 2004).

Within the context of therapy it is important to hold space to process what a woman in recovery may desire in terms of an intimate partner relationship and engage in therapeutic processing related to relational, emotional, or historical barriers and how to move through those effectively. Therapeutic space allows room to deal with competing concerns such as medication effects impacting libido, problems with sexual functioning, communication with an intimate partner, birth control, and boundary setting.

Identity

Identity issues are also important for clinicians to address when it comes to the relationship needs of women with SMI (Chernomas et al., 2000). Much of the literature indicates that women have some challenges with identity after experiencing an SMI. One qualitative study indicated that people felt a loss of self and had specific concerns about parenting, identity, and perceptions of normality (Wisdom, Bruce, Saedi, Weis, & Green, 2008). Given that women frequently connect some of their identity to their roles such as being a mother, a friend, a caregiver, or an intimate partner, it is crucial to explore and process the experience of mental illness and how this changes relational dynamics as they think about their identity.

Women have shared that contemplating having a child can feel painful and can shift their thoughts about personal identity (Anderson, 2014). Some women report that it has been difficult to process that life can be meaningful without having a child (Anderson, 2014). The narrative literature and the use of narrative therapy also indicates hope for returning to one's former self, developing new identities, or reconciling the self (Wisdom et al., 2008). Offering messages of strength, hope, and encouragement may aid in this process, and providers can emphasize that a meaningful life can be developed and be defined with one's own perspective and voice rather than being predetermined by others.

Women can become savvy cultural negotiators of the diverse challenges they experience due to stigma, isolation, and symptoms. Some women may seek out new roles, such as peer advocacy, which may provide new meaning and purpose for their experiences. Such new endeavors may be of particular interest to women with SMI and may encourage the use and development of versatile relational skills.

Group Strategies

Some group approaches might be beneficial to the relationship needs of women with SMI, such as a social skills training group or an acceptance and commitment therapy group (Bach, Gaudiano, Hayes, & Herbert, 2013; Bellack, Mueser, Gingerich, & Agresta, 2014). A social skills group can help target specific benchmarks and enhance interpersonal skills such as asking someone on a date, saying "no" to someone respectfully, maintaining healthy boundaries, and giving feedback. This type of group is conducted in a role-playing style that can be enjoyable and create a fun learning environment. An acceptance and commitment therapy group can help women in recovery with mindfulness and acceptance of some of their challenges. It also can increase their capacity to make progress toward their goals and identify the values they have as a person and in relationships. Both of these therapies have strong empirical support.

Support groups that may be helpful for family members of women with SMI include Family-to-Family or a family support group developed by the National Alliance on Mental Illness (NAMI). These groups can help family members learn more about managing their affect and their roles, and how to best support the individual in recovery (NAMI, 2019). Family-to-Family is considered an evidence-based practice by the Substance Abuse and Mental Health Services Administration (SAMHSA) and is taught by trained family members of individuals who experience mental illness. Family-to-Family helps develop strategies related to increasing understanding and psychoeducation, caregiving, problem-solving skills, supportiveness, and communication capabilities (NAMI, 2019). Significant changes can then occur in a family member's ability to solve problems and cope in the context of having a loved one with mental illness.

Psychoeducation should be assessed regarding its appropriateness for each individual and family (Dixon et al., 2000). The assessment should consider the extent and quality of the family and the individual involved, the interest level, the presence of outcomes that can be identified as goals, and whether family psychoeducation is preferred to other options to achieve similar outcomes.

Lefley (2009) provides a good overview of different modalities of intervention and work with families and puts them in perspective. According to this overview, family psychoeducation (Leff, 2005) focuses on illness management and problem solving and can reduce relapse and rehospitalization rates. It also can reduce symptoms, increase the employability of people with SMI, help caregivers to reduce family burden, and improve coping with the fact that a loved one has a mental illness. Family education is a multi-family group modality, led by professionally trained peers, that provides education, support, and illness management; it has been shown to increase family well-being irrespective of patient outcomes (for an overview see Lefley, 2009).

Of course, family therapy in general can be helpful and is a modality for addressing family dysfunction or challenges; its focus is to help the family function better, building on family systems theory (Lefley, 2009). Family consultation, another modality for resolving family-defined problems, involves a more infrequent advisor than ongoing therapist role. Psychoeducational support groups are multi-family groups that involve education and illness-management strategies. The literature indicates that psychoeducational support groups use group sharing to improve coping and also use advocacy to give mastery over one's own life, which in turn has been shown to improve family and patient well-being. A book that may be helpful for the family member of those with mental illness or those working with a family is Lieberman's (2009) *Recovery from Disability: Manual of Psychiatric Rehabilitation*. Lieberman also has many educational resources, videos, and diverse formats that are useful to support families.

Resources

Women with SMI can be supported to identify and connect to resources. For women in difficult housing or living situations, it may be helpful to identify different housing options or connect the woman with agencies that can help her navigate these complexities. This can be quite complicated if the woman has a conservator, is in a hospital setting, or is on public assistance. However, advocating for the woman and helping connect her to appropriate social resources may help her solve the problems she is experiencing in relationships (e.g., interpersonal violence, the need for greater independence/autonomy, enhanced boundaries in relationships, homelessness). Providers can aid the woman to develop financial, educational, or occupational goals and related steps to take so she has choice and boundaries in relationships.

Some models of increasing social support and friendship include intentional friendship as an adjunct to mental health services. One model of intentional friendship fosters relationships with community volunteers and has been found to be an effective method for increasing social support, with increases shown in subjective well-being and decreases in psychiatric symptoms (McCorkle, Rogers, Dunn, Lyass, & Wan, 2008). An intentional friend can serve as a mechanism to build social interactions and friendship skills over time. Creating natural supports and friendships would be ideal, but formation may initially need support through such mechanisms as intentional friendship.

Clinicians can also think of ways to create natural supports and develop friendships in the community. If the woman is interested in a certain community activity, how could she meet other people who are interested in those same activities? Examples include community book groups, town or library movie nights, music venues, political gatherings, and athletic activities such as road races, free yoga events, or a local gym class. Many of these could be identified in the newspaper or online. Women with SMI could also use social media to meet others with similar interests. Such activities can help women develop a meaningful life and friendships based on personal goals, interests, and hobbies, rather than based on a relationship developed within the context of seeking mental health services. These activities and friendship also may help the woman develop a sense of valued social roles, which have been identified as conducive to recovery (Davidson et al., 2009).

Other considerations to support women in recovery should include access to adequate transportation and childcare. Case management can help with these resources as well as parent education and support groups, respite services, and child resource needs (Nicholson & Biebel, 2002). The online parenting resource worksheet *Parenting with a Mental Illness: Programs and Resources* could be downloaded for free (UPENN Collaborative on Community Integration, 2019). This same organization provides a *Parenting Toolkit* and online training and curriculum for parenting with a psychiatric disability, which is modified for parenting at different developmental stages (TU Collaborative, 2019). Mental health systems should also prioritize individual and family services for women with children who can be served simultaneously with these services.

CONCLUSION

Women are socialized to value relationships, and those with SMI have unique relational concerns and experiences that need acknowledgment and attention within the clinical literature. Women face many pressures from society, families, and friends and as a result of their own internalized oppressive beliefs about their identity. It is crucial to explore the relationship goals and dynamics of women with SMI and to address their relational needs as they work on their recovery.

CLINICAL STRATEGIES

- Inquire about the relationships that are important for women with SMI as they envision working toward their dreams and goals in life.
- Attempt to identify relationship difficulties and the resources that could help support a woman with her relationship goals. This could include better boundaries, more autonomy, a deeper relationship, problem-solving skills, conflict-resolution skills, communication skills, and assertiveness training. Resources such as DBT, behavioral family therapy, and empowerment therapy (Linehan, 2014; Mueser & Glynn, 1996; Worell & Remer, 2003) may be helpful in these areas.
- Use person-centered treatment planning (Tondora et al., 2014) to identify achievable and measurable goals the woman has and relational supports to meet those goals.
- Explore a woman's goals around dating and partnership. Identify any past, current, or future challenges with these relational goals. Process these challenges and learn how the woman may prefer to work on such challenges.
- Always remember to assess for any experiences of trauma or interpersonal violence. Appropriately engage in a detailed trauma assessment and connect the woman to the appropriate resources, such as specific psychotherapy interventions, behavioral interventions, and systemic supports like trauma-informed care.
- Normalize the experiences of women with SMI by sharing what is known about women with similar experiences such as (1) common challenges and competing demands with navigating one's recovery and desire to have an intimate partner, (2) medication side effects impacting libido or sexual functioning, (3) value of healthy familial support, (4) differences in relationships that women have felt before and after the SMI diagnosis, (5) feelings during and about motherhood, and (6) custody rights of women with SMI.
- Identify resources to develop dating skills, such as assertiveness training. Explore hobbies or social clubs in which connection to others can occur. Identify safety strategies. Support exploration of social media resources, which may be useful for finding dating partners.
- Identify resources that may be helpful for the continuum of experiences, including motherhood. This could include many things such as books, online platforms, mothers' support groups, or other formats. Identify health care that can be extremely supportive during pregnancy and postpartum months. Provide collaborative care and connection to local resources such as parenting groups, breastfeeding classes, and birthing classes.
- Emphasize what choice a woman has in her relationships and how she can exercise her options in those relationships.

- Support women in developing relationships with friends who can be supportive of each other and their recovery. Identify what types of friend relationships they want to develop or deepen and the mechanisms to do so.

DISCUSSION QUESTIONS

1. The mental health field has long ignored the interests of women with SMI and their desires for an intimate partner. Their sexual needs have been denied, and deemed pathological if expressed. How do you think these biases developed in our culture? What contributed to them? What can our culture and systems of care do to support women in their interests in intimate relationships?
2. What rights to autonomous choice do you believe a woman with SMI should have? What about when she has been hospitalized against her will due to suicidality and voices telling her to also hurt others? What about when she has a conservator of person and estate?
3. How can our training institutions provide better education about the unique relational needs of women? How can these issues be incorporated into how women with SMI are conceptualized in terms of the challenges they are experiencing and the ways in which the mental health field should partner with them?

ACTIVITIES

The following activity has been developed to provide an educational experience about how we as a society might be socialized to act out gender and how that has an impact on women with SMI. In groups of three, discuss the topics and share as an entire group two or three takeaway topics that surfaced as part of this discussion.

1. In Western culture, what expectations are often put on women regarding motherhood? Think about this in terms of the following women (some of the bullet points may serve as brainstorming offshoots):
   - A woman who cannot have children
   - A woman who chooses not to have children
   - A woman who gives up her children.
   Consider a situation in which a mother does something that hurts a child. How would we react compared to when a father does this?
2. What are the sociocultural messages women receive about expectations for caring for disabled family members or older family members? What

if one cannot complete those tasks or finds them too burdensome? How
are these messages different with factors such as:
- Race/ethnicity
- National origin
- Socioeconomic status
- Ability status
- Educational status.

3. Identify any immediate biases you may hold (either implicit or explicit)
that may come up when you think about the rights of those with SMI to
have an intimate partner relationship. Use some of these ideas to start
your conversation:
- An individual wants to start a relationship on an inpatient
psychiatric unit
- An individual wants to find a partner to have a baby but is having
ongoing suicidality and cyclical hospitalization

4. What ethical issues come up as you think about the desire and right for
women with SMI to have choice as it relates to their intimate partner
relationships, family members, and friendships? Thinking about the
following situations may help this discussion:
- When an individual has a conservator or is involuntarily hospitalized
- When a woman wants to parent and keep children in her custody but
may not be able to at the current time
- When a woman continues to return to a relationship with domestic
violence, which spurs a cycle of rehospitalization and trauma.

Relationship Structuring Worksheet

People in Your Life	Quality of Relationship	Goals	Steps
Ex: Friends: Joyce	*Supportive*	*Go to movies*	*Text an invite*
Ex: Intimate Partner	*Conflicted*	*Communicate better*	*Set aside time to talk on weekend*
Family:			
Community:			
Children/Caregiving:			
Friends:			
Intimate Partner:			
School/Work/ Volunteer:			

5

Work and Class Among Women with Serious Mental Illness

Work gives meaning and structure to life, and can bring financial security along with a steady source of income. While women with serious mental illness (SMI) typically want to work, this desire is often frustrated by obstacles. Symptoms and stigma can interfere with attaining and sustaining competitive employment. A major mental health problem can also get in the way of acquiring the education needed to meet job requirements. Then there are the problems women have faced as a gender to achieve equity in wages, on top of expectations to carry out unpaid domestic labor within the home. Adding to all this is the fact that people with SMI often have low incomes, either due to the SMI interfering with employment, or as a result of the effects of poverty on mental health.

Yet there are few published studies on the topics of work and class for women with SMI. In our conversations with leaders in the field of psychiatric rehabilitation, they have confirmed that little to no research has been conducted on women with SMI in the area of work in particular (K. Mueser, personal communication, March 26, 2018; E. S. Rogers, personal communication, March 27, 2018). To fill this gap in the literature, we will focus on issues of work and class for women with SMI in this chapter. We will review the literature on issues of work and mental health for people with SMI. We will also cover research on the effects of poverty on mental health for these populations. Several case narratives from a qualitative study on women with SMI will illuminate relevant themes, followed by clinical strategies, and future research directions.

WOMEN AND WORK

A discussion of the mental health challenges posed to women in general in work is warranted at the outset of a discussion of those faced by women with SMI. Given the workaholic culture of the Western world, one might assume that work would be a source of psychological distress for women (and men) in general, not just for women with SMI. However, research has demonstrated that there are a number of benefits of employment for women's mental health under positive working conditions. Among the benefits of work to women are boosts in mental health; reductions in depression and anxiety; and a sense of control, power, and pride (Bildt & Michélsen, 2002; Repetti, Matthews, & Waldron, 1989; Rosenfield, 1989). The factors that tend to worsen mental health among working women include jobs with high levels of job strain, imbalances between effort and reward, job insecurity, and low levels of decision-making power and social support (Stansfeld & Candy, 2006). In this section, we will examine specific variables that affect women's mental health in the workplace, including family roles, work control, social support, and gender dynamics in the workplace.

Family Roles

Family gender dynamics appear to be a key variable that impacts the mental health of women who work. Researchers have found that the strain of multiple work roles both inside and outside of the home poses negative consequences to health and employment (Perrone, Wright, & Jackson, 2009; Repetti et al., 1989). Mental and physical health risks are particularly high for women with heavy job demands, young children, and husbands who avoid domestic labor. Women appear to cope with the stress of a dual-career couple by taking part-time or less challenging jobs, or even leaving the working world altogether (Woods, 1985). Much of this older research remains true decades later.

The homemaker role has been studied in some depth in relation to mental health. In a review of the literature, it appears that these women often have worse mental health (Frech & Damaske, 2012; Repetti et al., 1989; Rosenfield, 1989). However, the inverse is true when women aren't working outside the home due to mental health problems; this has particular implications for women with SMI. Furthermore, one study found that unemployed women took meaning from the caretaking role, and this buffered the effect of unemployment on their mental health, in contrast to unemployed men (Artazcoz, Benach, Borrell, & Cortès, 2004).

In general, research studies have shown that employed women are less anxious and depressed, or at least not more depressed than unemployed women, particularly if they have partners who help with any domestic labor responsibilities at home (Frech & Damaske, 2012; Repetti et al., 1989). In addition, the income and power gained from working outside the home might enhance the mental health benefits of work for women (Repetti et al., 1989; Rosenfield, 1989). However, these studies have suggested that in some cases, women may use unhealthy behaviors (e.g., alcohol abuse) to cope with work stress, just as men do.

Women may encounter a higher risk of depression and symptom chronicity due to low socioeconomic status (SES) and higher stressors, termed the "double burden" of work and home demands (Frech & Damaske, 2012; Muntaner, Eaton, Miech, & O'Campo, 2004). Arlie Hochschild famously named this phenomenon "the second shift" (Hochschild & Machung, 2003). This concept refers to the period of domestic labor (e.g., childcare, cooking, cleaning) that women face when coming home from their job, their first "shift." Levels of cortisol—the stress hormone—appear to decrease for men when they return home from work but remain spiked for women as a result of household chores. This double burden has been found to be worse for women who live in a state with a high level of income inequality (Muntaner et al., 2004). New mothers with lower income levels also tend to have high rates of postpartum depression, likely due to financial anxiety and a lack of resources needed for support.

Work Control

Several studies have investigated the effects of work control on women's mental health. Rosenfield (1989) found that women who worked outside the home exchange low control in one area for another, such as a lack of decision-making power in the family. A combination of a work environment with a lack of control, high work demand, and low power for the female worker could increase her symptoms of anxiety and depression (Frech & Damaske, 2012; Rosenfield, 1989).

In another study, Lennon and Rosenfield (1992) found that the effect of family demands on the mental health of women was moderated by level of control at work. Married women with good job control were less distressed than housewives and working women with a poor sense of control and autonomy at work. The authors of this study suggested that a strong coping ability could help women to acquire work with more control, leading to higher levels of well-being. More recent research also shows that having control in the workplace diminishes job stress (Rivera-Torres, Araque-Padilla, & Montero-Simó, 2013). However, these multiple work and coping factors may be difficult to navigate for women who are also managing the symptoms of an SMI.

Social Support

Social support is another factor that influences women's well-being in the workplace. For example, physical health is improved for employed women if they have positive attitudes toward their work. The connection between health and work is further bolstered by the presence of supportive coworkers and supervisors, given the expansion of one's social network offered by work (Repetti et al., 1989; Rivera-Torres et al., 2013). This is called the "healthy worker effect" (Repetti et al., 1989).

In addition to low social support, subclinical depression and alcohol use appear to be affected by a number of problematic conditions that women often face in the workplace (Bildt & Michélsen, 2002). These difficult work conditions include shift work and temporary work, as well as low levels of work pride, stimulation, or opportunities for professional and educational development. Women may become increasingly strained if they have to balance domestic labor in their homes with shift work.

Gendered Workplaces

Jobs that are traditionally gendered also appear to impact women's mental health, given that women's jobs tend to have low status, and therefore are high in stress and low in control (Bildt & Michélsen, 2002). Female-dominated workplaces include jobs in hospitality, administrative support, and caregiving (Milner, King, LaMontagne, Bentley, & Kavanagh, 2018). Women also tend to have more demanding positions with less power than men in these professions, worsening their mental health (Rosenfield, 1989). In contrast, men's mental health tends to improve in male-dominated workplaces (Milner et al., 2018).

While many of the key studies on women, work, and mental health are older (and heterocentric), the findings of these studies continue to apply today. Many women still feel forced to decide between advancing their partner's careers or their own, and managing childcare, posing considerable stress. And for women who are vulnerable to mental illness, demands of the home and workplace may push their mental health over the edge.

WORK AND GENDER AMONG PEOPLE WITH SMI

Clearly, women as a gender have to reckon with many strains on their mental health when it comes to work. For women with SMI, there is even more to juggle when it comes to stigma and symptoms that could interfere with work. However, while there is a substantive body of literature on work and people with SMI (see Crowther, Marshall, Bond, & Huxley, 2001, and Frederick & VanderWeele, 2019, for reviews), little of this research has examined the impact of gender. Among the few vocational rehabilitation studies on people with SMI that have included the variable of gender in the analyses, little to no relationship has been found between gender and work (Kirsh, 2000; Mowbray et al., 1995). For example, one vocational rehabilitation study of 275 participants in Boston found no gender differences—this was in the area of social outcomes between employed and unemployed participants (Rogers et al., 1991). However, a Scottish survey of schizophrenia found that men were less likely to be employed (McCreadie, 1982). This finding was replicated in other studies in the United States (Beiser et al., 1994) and in the United Kingdom (Harrison et al., 1996). These results suggest that women with SMI may have unique sources of resilience in achieving employment, a point that requires further study.

A related study on supported employment for adults with developmental disabilities found that supervisors perceived women to be more socially appropriate at work (Olson, Cioffi, Yovanoff, & Mank, 2000). However, the women were still limited by more traditionally gendered jobs, fewer hours, and lower wages than men. This confirmed previous research that women earn less money and are less likely to have competitive employment. More research is needed to explore gender differences in supported employment for people with SMI.

To address this gap, one of the authors (Mizock) worked with several graduate students to analyze the data on work in her qualitative study with women with SMI. They published those results in the *Journal of Vocational Rehabilitation* (Mizock, Aitken, & LaMar, 2019). Themes generated from the qualitative interviews are listed in Table 5.1.

The final two themes in particular demonstrated the resilience of women with SMI in finding meaningful work outside of the conventional employment sphere, overcoming barriers they face in the working world.

Other qualitative research on work in both men and women with SMI found that a number of behavioral strategies appeared to help them function well at work and in general (Glynn et al., 2010). These coping mechanisms included medication adherence, health behaviors (exercise, sleep, nutrition), spiritual activities, living with a pet or someone else, and involvement in the recovery movement. They also attributed gains in their work and general functioning to avoiding alcohol and substance use, travel, crowds, and isolating behaviors.

Table 5.1 QUALITATIVE THEMES PERTAINING TO WORK EXPERIENCES OF WOMEN WITH SMI ($N = 20$)

Themes	Definitions
Work Drain	Tendency for workplace stress to psychologically deplete women with SMI, often exacerbating their symptoms.
Symptom Visibility	Challenges women with SMI may have in hiding their symptoms at work, often leading to adverse consequences.
Work Disclosure	The dilemma faced by the women with SMI regarding whether and how much to disclose their mental health challenges to supervisors and coworkers.
Inconsistent Work	Difficulties women with SMI face in maintaining steady employment, periodically losing jobs or being forced to quit because of mental health challenges.
Nontraditional Work	Phenomenon in which women with SMI adapt to challenges posed by their symptoms and external adversity and find meaningful work by starting their own businesses, engaging in gender non-conforming work (e.g., carpenter, bouncer), or redefining traditional work roles (e.g., motherhood).
Work Assets	Resilience factors that women with SMI demonstrate in employment experiences, including community resources, personal contacts, and personal strengths.

From Mizock, Aitken, & LaMar (2019). Reprinted with permission from *Journal of Vocational Rehabilitation* © 2019.

CLASS

There are clear financial implications of work barriers for women with SMI. These women may have lower incomes as a result of symptoms and stigma, and can grapple with extreme poverty. In turn, poverty can have a devastating effect on their physical and mental health. Poverty has been linked to harmful consequences like stress, pessimism, helplessness, and insomnia (Adler, Epel, Castellazo, & Ickovics, 2000). Hence, there is a bidirectional relationship between mental health and wealth for women with SMI, as illustrated in Figure 5.1. In this section, we will review the literature on the impact of class, SES, and poverty on the mental health of women in general, and those with SMI in particular.

Women and Poverty

Belle (1990) conducted a key literature review of the effects of poverty on the mental health of women. In sum, women appear to be disproportionately affected by poverty, and poverty has a primary effect on mental health. Lower-income women have a higher incidence of mental illness. Women's elevated rates of poverty have been connected to a number of sociocultural and economic changes, such as a growing lack of partners in families headed by women, affordable childcare, child support, government subsidies to low-income families, and housing for mothers.

Women with young children are the most likely renters to experience eviction, and this often fuels a downward spiral in terms of finances and mental health.

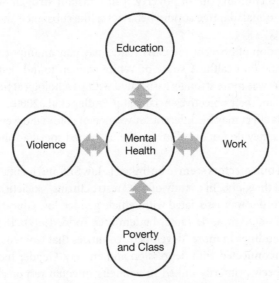

Figure 5.1 Bidirectional relationships with variables pertaining to work, class, and mental health

In Matthew Desmond's book (2016) *Evicted*, he documented the difficulties that housing problems pose to these women:

> One in two recently evicted mothers reports multiple symptoms of clinical depression, double the rate of similar mothers who were not forced from their homes. Even after years pass, evicted mothers are less happy, energetic, and optimistic than their peers. When several patients committed suicide in the days leading up to their eviction, a group of psychiatrists published a letter in *Psychiatric Services*, identifying eviction as a "significant precursor of suicide." The letter emphasized that none of the patients were facing homelessness, leading the psychiatrists to attribute the suicides to eviction itself. "Eviction must be considered a traumatic rejection," they wrote, "a denial of one's most basic human needs, and an exquisitely shameful experience." Suicides attributed to evictions and foreclosures doubled between 2005 and 2010, years when housing costs soared. (p. 298)

In his compelling work, Desmond adds that eviction can lead to employment instability and job loss because of its negative impact on job performance due to disabling stress.

Intersectional disparities add to these economic problems for women. For example, Black and Latina women are at particular risk of poverty, as well as eviction (Belle, 1990; Desmond, 2016). High rates of depression have also been found among unemployed low-income women without childcare help. Impoverished women tend to have higher rates of exposure to violence and crime, yet their coping strategies for dealing with the mental health effects of poverty may be limited by a sense of powerlessness in the face of the relentless obstacles to climbing out of poverty. This constant struggle with no end in sight can lead to maladaptive coping behaviors, like substance abuse and eating disorders.

One's perception of poverty and class status may play an important role in the effects of income on health. A study of White women found that their subjective social status was more strongly associated with psychological functioning and health rather than their objective social status (Adler et al., 2000). It is important to note that this effect may be different for women of color who were not included in this study, as they do not benefit from the unearned social advantage of White privilege.

A number of other factors seem to be linked to low SES and mental health among women around the globe. In a study of five "restructuring" societies, the presence of a mental disorder was associated with female gender, low education, older age, and poverty (Patel, Araya, de Lima, Ludemir, & Todd, 1999). These results extend previous findings in more "developed" countries that women's experience of poverty is interconnected with depression and anxiety. Gender inequities across cultures have been primarily linked to women's unequal responsibilities in uncompensated family caretaking, harkening back to our earlier discussion of the invisibility of domestic labor.

Adding to the concern about women's poverty rates around the world are the high rates of violence toward women (Patel et al., 1999). The mental health consequences of violence include depression, anxiety, post-traumatic stress disorder (PTSD), dissociation disorders, somatization disorders, sexual disorders, and self-harming behaviors (Fischbach & Herbert, 1997). Thus, another bidirectional relationship (captured in Figure 5.1) can be found in the link between victimization and negative mental health outcomes.

Poverty and Mental Health

Low SES can be both a cause *and* an outcome of mental illness. People from low-income families appear to have been diagnosed with a high rate of mental disorders during adolescence in particular (Miech et al., 1999). The link between SES and SMI has been explained by "social causation" models (stress causes low SES) and "social selection" models (downward mobility occurs with genetic predisposition) (Dohrenwend et al., 1992). Dohrenwend and colleagues conducted a large study with Israelis to investigate these issues. The social causation model explained the higher rates of depression in women compared to men. However, the social selection model captured the relationship between SES and schizophrenia, which was often genetic and also led to economic challenges. These diverging models reflect differences in the mechanics of the relationship between poverty and mental health.

Poverty is a key stressor for people with SMI. U.S. Census data indicate that there is a higher rate of SMI among low-SES people (Ware & Goldfinger, 1997). A third model, the "social-economic stress model" (Hudson, 2005), explains this phenomenon. In this model, the stressors of poverty, unemployment, and housing problems are understood to contribute to the onset of SMI.

Perese (2007) provided an overview of some of the barriers to recovery posed by stigma, poverty, and victimization for people with SMI. For one, stigma can interfere with health insurance coverage and result in difficulties qualifying for public assistance programs, like Medicaid and social security income (SSI). People with SMI might not meet criteria for these programs or might encounter barriers to follow-through, like symptoms or homelessness. Moreover, stigma can lead to work discrimination and employment problems, interfering with acquiring safe housing.

In an earlier study, Perese (1997) found the primary unmet needs reported by people with SMI pertained to identity, safety, and money. In this study, most people with SMI didn't have enough money for their basic needs for the month, including housing and transportation. Unmet needs appear to be connected to lower quality of life and higher hospitalization rates (Perese, 1997). Poverty can also lead to social withdrawal among people with SMI due to the economic demands of social participation. Furthermore, there is a higher risk of victimization in cases of poverty, particularly among women and homeless people with SMI, all of whom are vulnerable to financial exploitation. Thus, researchers have argued that poverty is a central factor in the lack of community and social integration among people with SMI (Yanos et al., 2001).

Based on this literature, we can presume that the economic challenges of people with SMI may interfere with work through a lack of financial resources that chip away at mental health and one's stability in the community. In contrast, women with SMI with more financial resources may have more educational opportunities, mental health supports, and access to safe housing—all factors that can boost mental health.

We present the following three case narratives to explore issues of work and class among women with SMI, topics that have been missing in the literature. These stories are developed from research interviews with women with SMI and were selected because they featured issues of class, work, and gender. The case narratives include an overview of the person's demographic and family background, mental health history, and experiences with work and class. Applications to clinical work will be presented based on the lived experiences of these women.

CASE NARRATIVES

Case 1: Dora

"Dora" is an Italian American, Catholic, bisexual woman in her 60s. Dora identifies as a person in recovery and has been attending therapy on and off since age 25. She has diagnoses of major depression and PTSD, among others, including borderline personality disorder, bipolar disorder, and anxiety disorder. She has a master's degree in education and taught high school early in her career. However, her work was derailed by chronic pain and mental health problems.

When asked about her class background, Dora stated, "I guess I grew up working class. But truth be told, some of the time we were really poor. But it was never defined that way . . . We were working class, but my dad had a gambling problem which made us sometimes poor." As an adult, Dora identifies her class differently: "Now I'm technically low income, I suppose, because of my disability circumstances. But I'm a very educated person with a master's degree and have been a professional, so I sort of cross classes." She added, "It's not at all clear for a lot of people and for me . . . I used to say to friends years ago that [my family] crossed the class border and we had feet in both sides, because we grew up poor or working class and then we got educated . . . Then I got poor again because of my health issues. But you don't lose everything you gained when you upwardly mobile in educational and other ways."

Interestingly, in the author's (Mizock's) qualitative research with women with SMI, many of the participants did not provide a one-word answer when asked about their class. Instead, a story emerged that often involved a middle-class beginning with a transition to a state of poverty after the development of SMI. Mental illness tended to stall the start of their careers or interfere with the pursuit of a career altogether. And like other women with SMI, poverty associated with Dora's employment problems stemmed from her mental and physical health problems, leading to additional risk factors. She explained:

> I was at risk for homelessness. And if it wasn't for the fact that the universe just sort of adjusted itself at the time I needed it to, I would have been homeless a number of years ago. I experienced some discrimination at my job. Not because of my mental illness, but because of some of my physical disabilities. And as a result, my depression got really bad at that time. Although that was the beginning of it getting really worse and PTSD sort of getting—coming to a head. I ended up leaving that job because of how it affected me mentally. And so, I ended up with no income and unable to work for quite a while. I would have been homeless at that time but it just so happened that the apartment complex that I lived in serendipitously converted to an affordable housing cooperative. It happened at the same time so I didn't lose my housing, because [of] the change to rent being based on your income, which wasn't the case before. So I was able to live here and pay very, very, very little. And so I didn't become homeless. . . . I did have to completely do a switch from my professional life to getting food stamps, and getting different services. Going to food pantries and soup kitchens.

Despite Dora's difficulty maintaining traditional work, she continued to find meaningful work that added purpose to her day, a valuable alternative for women with SMI who can't maintain traditional employment:

> I try to do a lot of things to keep me going. And I do artwork, which is what's kept me surviving through everything, especially since when I had lost the job and being discriminated against and all that stuff happened and my life fell apart . . . When I was first experiencing all these problems at that job, I used to go home, and I would sit up all night beading. Just sort of de-stressing. And then I was wearing some of my creations. And people started asking me about my work, you know, asking me where I got the jewelry. I said I made it, and people started asking me to make them things. So I didn't really realize that I had this talent until people started asking for specific things. And I would go home and try to create it, and discovered that I had an eye for color and design. So when I lost the teaching job completely, I eked out a new living with the jewelry business. I did open studios and arts and crafts shows, and art shows and stuff like that . . . When I fell down the stairs on my spine, which was about six years ago, I stopped because I couldn't even sit long enough to do anything for over two years. But then I got back into it a little bit.

Dora found work in other creative interests:

> I've also periodically been painting, even though I don't know much about painting. I had some people like my work, and I was invited to sell my work

on this website that this person in [my town] started for homeless and disabled artists. Actually, you can go on there and see some of my work. So I really still know nothing about painting. But periodically I come up with something that looks good. In fact, I've been painting while talking to you even though I'm just doodling and doing nothing. Just to keep me calm . . . I also learned to be really good with money so I could survive with very little and be well. . . . Yeah, I think my creativity helps me a lot, too. Not just in the work and the stuff I do, but just being creative. Just being resourceful.

Dora demonstrated resilience in managing poverty and employment by accessing her creativity and pursuing meaningful, flexible work. She was able to become an entrepreneur as a craftsperson, which provided some income along with a sense of pride and industriousness as a solo business owner.

Dora wasn't alone. Other women with SMI in these interviews described navigating employment challenges by working for themselves or for friends, or pursuing meaningful work when possible, even if unpaid, as we will see in the following case vignettes.

Case 2: Sally

"Sally" is a lesbian, Jewish American woman in her late 40s. She has been diagnosed with severe depression, an anxiety disorder, and epilepsy. She has a family history of depression, bipolar disorder, autism, and compulsive gambling. When asked about how she identified her class background, she did not provide a closed-ended answer. Rather, another story ensued: "I see myself as working class . . . That's what I spent most of my adult life as. My mother and my father and my grandmother . . . all worked. Well, my mother didn't work until . . . I went to school until I was about five or six."

Sally's family finances changed when her father died:

My feelings are that our income level probably crashed, or the money coming in. I mean, I'm sure [my mother] found a way to live off death benefits and stuff. And she got survivor benefits for me and my brother for a while. But looking back on this much later, I think we were probably middle class while my dad was alive. And I'm guessing that we didn't stay there. And I've always had, I mean I worked in health care—which is a pretty blue-color job—most of my adult life.

Like Dora and many other women with SMI, employment and economic problems led to risks of homelessness, as she had "been on the edge of homelessness, but I have never quite been homeless." Because of her family resources, she was able to keep from becoming fully homeless.

Sally explained how her identity as a lesbian also posed risk to her financial wellness:

I think when I came out in the [19]80s, the understanding was if you were a lesbian then you were pretty much going to be poor . . . That's probably not as true today. But I think when I came out, that was pretty much a given, that you were going to be poor. And gay men were poorer than straight men . . . It was like a hierarchy. If you were any kind of minority on top of it, you were going to be poorer . . . And that was the way it was going to be, and there really wasn't much you could do about it. So I was kind of expecting to be poor.

In fact, Sally's career choice was influenced by a desire to find acceptance around her sexuality:

I guess I kind of gravitated towards jobs where it wouldn't matter as much, or tried to. And it turned out that there were a lot of gays and lesbians that work in health care. They didn't care as much. They cared about could you do the work, and they didn't care as much about if you were gay or not. And I guess the money was better than some fields. And the health care was good. And somehow, I guess we instinctively knew that. But at least the money was good at the beginning. Then the economy tanked . . . Everyone started earning less . . .

But, I first went into health care because I thought the only skills I had when I left college was doing direct care with people like my brother [who had severe autism]. After I had the more standard jobs of working in a restaurant . . . The corporate world thing was just beginning to kind of get started, and I knew that I couldn't deal with that. And I knew that I couldn't deal with calling people and begging them for money, like some of my friends did. I knew that I couldn't do that, and that I would hate that, and that it would eat my soul, and I just couldn't do it. So, you know, this is what I thought would be the only job. And it turned out that I was good at it. And I did it for quite a long time.

But you know, it wasn't a terrible job. As long as you did what you were supposed to. And you were kind of left alone, too, which was another advantage. Compared to a lot of jobs, you're largely left alone as long as you did what you were supposed to do and nothing was horribly wrong . . . Because if you were out, it was a big deal, you couldn't necessarily work with kids . . . And not that I particularly wanted to work with kids. Yeah, there were professions you couldn't really enter. You know, if someone found out or suspected, you could get fired. There weren't—initially at least—there weren't job protections and stuff.

The stress of Sally's job began to affect her mental health and her ability to work, and she left her job:

I stopped work by the time I got a diagnosis. So I wasn't really thinking of myself as a woman with a mental health issue, until I was pretty much stopped working. . . . I was having sleep issues. I think I was definitely having depression issues. I mean, I probably had been for quite a long time. There were some building issues. We had unionized at work and they were fucking with me. There were a lot of things going on. I was doing collective bargaining for 18 months and they were fucking with me at work. You know, there were all kinds of stuff going on. I had really burned myself out. My bosses were horrible people.

However, Sally found that her job had given her tools in her own mental health management:

Because I worked in health care, I learned to advocate for other people. I know a lot about bureaucracy and how to advocate for myself. It's not something we're taught. A lot of people learn or by accident know how to do it. If people never learn it, or you don't learn certain skills, then you're going to get fucked over more. You know, not told things that you need to know. Because we're not taught these things in our society. And some people are really good. My friend C--- is really good at resource gathering. She is even better than I am. But there is no guide to resource gathering for people, which there should be.

Sally also felt that her Jewish background had led others to make assumptions that she had more class privilege than she in fact did. She described the stereotype of

the whole thing that Jews control all the money in the world. But would I be living in [subsidized housing]. and getting on disability, and $11 in food stamps if we ran the world? I'd be getting a check. I'd be living in a mansion somewhere getting a check, you know? I'd own my own condo or my own house somewhere, and I'd be getting a check every month from "Jewish Inc." or something!

Sally was particularly attuned to issues of class, likely due to her identity as a lesbian and her awareness of issues of societal oppression. She spoke about mental health as knowing no class lines: "Mental health cuts across everything. Plus, 'crazies' are everywhere," she said in jest. "'Crazy' will cut across anything. Rich people are crazy. Poor people are crazy. Everyone has crazy people in their family. 'Crazy' doesn't care . . . Some people just hide it better, or have money to hide it. Or send people away."

Sally's story demonstrates the complex intersections of mental health, gender, sexual orientation, disability, class, and religion on the impact on financial wellness. As a result of intersectional stigma, she became particularly conscious of how oppression operates. Her experience also highlights how work stress could complicate the ability of a woman with SMI to remain employed. Moreover, family resources supported her in pursuing the education needed to attain competitive, paid work and prevent homelessness. Overall, Sally's case exemplifies how women with SMI learn to self-advocate and seek resources to manage their employment and financial needs.

Case 3: Loni

"Loni" is a White, heterosexual, Jewish woman of Greek and Bulgarian heritage in her mid-60. Her father was a chemical engineer and her mother worked as a housekeeper, becoming a bookkeeper later in life. She was diagnosed with bipolar disorder in her early 20s, as well as obsessive-compulsive disorder (OCD) when she was older. Her providers had some difficulty identifying her diagnosis, and she was in and out of hospitals for some time in her early adulthood. She graduated from college and became a secretary, a job that was later derailed by her OCD.

Like the previous women, Loni did not give a one-word answer when asked to identify her class: "My father had money and we had a very full house. I had a nanny. We went to good schools. But then my parents divorced, and I mostly lived with my mother in Queens. But I would say that was just a notch down—just middle class." Loni gained a half-brother after her mother remarried, who is her current guardian and manages her finances: "He is taking my money, and handling the rent, and trying to get all the worries out of my head so I have a nicer life. And I live in an assisted living building now, because I was in a hospital, and they wouldn't let me go home." While some people with SMI encounter power struggles with family who manage their finances, Loni feels she has a good relationship with this family member and finds his support with financial matters helpful.

Loni's work was complicated by the mental health problem and stigma she confronted at work: "I didn't know anybody else but me in the workplace who had a mental health problem. There was obviously only one. I was the only one declared, anyway." When asked if she was treated fairly at work, she replied:

> No . . . I'm much older than these new things that came in, like reasonable accommodations, like having a cot. I really got tired after lunch, and I really needed like an hour's sleep. And I found some place to sleep, and I would just disappear. But the big boss didn't like that at all. He said, "She's away from her desk too much." . . . I would come back very refreshed. I was a very good worker, but I just needed extra time. He just wanted to cut me down . . . because of these times. But actually when I was there, I was very productive, and I overproduced in order to cover so that nobody would be without work done. I asked the department to give me whatever work they had, like over spring break and all these breaks. I would just do it and be there till late and get there early in the morning and just do work.

Loni decided to seek the help of the union in response to this conflict with her supervisor: "My immediate boss wound up helping me because she had a child with Down's syndrome. She was like, 'When you're sick, you're sick. You can't help it.' . . . There was a fight about me. And I think she won.'"

Loni's story demonstrated how women with SMI might need accommodations in the workplace in order to perform their job. The understanding and support of a supervisor like Loni's can help to mitigate challenges in the workplace. Support from family members in managing financial concerns could also help build a safety net. Her story also demonstrates how women with SMI might overcompensate in the workplace by working harder and taking on extra work. The lack of rights for workers with psychiatric disabilities could clearly take a toll on the mental health of women with SMI.

UNDERSTANDING CLASS AND WORK FOR WOMEN WITH SMI

As shown in the case vignettes, women with SMI could experience their class backgrounds in a narrative manner. The common story involves a reduction in financial resources with the development of a mental illness. Those mental health challenges could further interfere with school and work. All of this could even lead to homelessness. Women with SMI from other marginalized groups might encounter even greater risks of poverty and stigma that could jeopardize their financial stability, like women of color or queer women. They may also face compounded barriers in education and work discrimination. On the other hand, women with SMI often demonstrate a number of resources and coping strategies to counterbalance these obstacles. They may find friends and family members to support their financial wellness and help them to handle financial resources.

It is important to acknowledge that the case narratives in this chapter featured all White women. While these cases selected from the study of women with SMI included particularly rich accounts of issues of class and work for women with SMI, there is much more to say about the class and work issues of women of color with SMI. Like Sally, racism poses a risk to financial wellness in a culture where race and class are stratified. White women carry unearned social advantages that can protect them from many hardships, such as the effects of systemic racism on financial and educational attainment. More research in this area could involve the resilience of low-income women with SMI who are women of color, sexual minorities, or transgender and gender diverse.

The literature review and case narratives show that women with SMI face unique challenges in work and finances. Clinicians can enhance women's awareness of any barriers or facilitators to work, education, and financial wellness and access to beneficial resources. (Table 5.2 lists work and financial challenges and supports among women with SMI.)

Specifically, clinicians might explore any issues of work discrimination related to intersectional stigma (or multiple levels of stigma and oppression) that a particular woman with SMI may encounter. Intersectional stigma could include experiences of sexism and mental illness stigma in the workplace, as well

Table 5.2. WORK AND FINANCIAL CHALLENGES AND SUPPORTS AMONG WOMEN
WITH SMI

Work and Financial Challenges	Work and Financial Supports
Intersectional stigma (sexism, mental illness stigma, racism, classism, homophobia, etc.)	Social network/capital
	Mental health services
	Flexible and nontraditional work
Traditional gender dynamics at work	Meaningful unpaid work
High-demand work/shift work	Supported employment/education and
Work discrimination/wage gap	vocational rehabilitation programs
Domestic labor demands/"second shift"	High-control/power/status work
Low-control/power/status work	Strong social support at work
Weak social support at work	Peer and advocacy jobs
Traditional gender dynamics	Source of income
Low income	Education
Educational barriers and discrimination	Stable, affordable, and safe housing
Housing barriers and discrimination	Trustworthy financial advisors
Financial exploiters	

as racism, classism, ableism, homophobia, and/or perhaps transphobia in the case of transgender and gender-diverse women with SMI. Clinicians can conduct the Women's Empowerment and Recovery-Oriented Care (WE-ROC) model (see Chapter 9) in which experiences with intersectional stigma are named and validated. This approach can help women with SMI feel empowered in managing intersectional stigma.

Clinicians can help women with SMI to access social capital in their support network. Licensed mental health providers in many states are mandated to report financial exploitation. Clinicians can help women with SMI to detect these warning signs in their relationships and family, and to seek help when needed. Clinicians can also invite women with SMI to tell the stories of their class background, witnessing the financial struggles that may have developed alongside the SMI. Alternatively, clinicians can raise awareness of the risks of poverty on the mental health of women with SMI they are working with.

Given that women with SMI are vulnerable to work discrimination, clinicians can help them to advocate and access worker protections. Clinicians might also refer women with SMI to a supported employment or vocational rehabilitation program in order to receive specialized services in this area. Additionally, supported education programs are in development that could help women with SMI return to school to learn new skills that enhance their job competitiveness. Case management can be used with women with SMI in order to investigate public sources of assistance such as Medicaid and SSI, as well as housing programs. These resources could provide an economic safety net to diminish the adverse effects of poverty on women's mental health and prevent homelessness.

Clinicians can assess the various factors in the workplace of women with SMI that might negatively impact their work, such as traditional gender dynamics, high work demands, shift work, and other inflexible arrangements. Providers can help women to explore accommodations in the workplace and to become aware of their rights in this area, enlisting legal services when needed. They can also coach women with SMI to bolster their support network in the workplace by forming alliances with coworkers and supervisors. Clinicians also need to assist women with SMI to navigate issues related to disclosure of their SMI in the workplace, and related issues of stigma, privacy, and worker protections.

These cases reveal the possibility that women with SMI could seek flexible and nontraditional work options. Clinicians can encourage women with SMI to network with friends for jobs, become self-employed, or pursue other kinds of flexible paid or unpaid work and volunteer opportunities that add structure and purpose to the day. Other sources of meaningful work might also include peer specialist jobs that allow women with SMI to draw from their experiences to help others.

Based on the literature review on gender and work, clinicians should encourage women with SMI to find work with high control, power, and status as much as possible in order to offer the greatest mental health benefit. Clinicians can assess the degree to which women with SMI might encounter domestic labor expectations that could add stress or strain, such as child, partner, or elder caretaker demands. Some women with SMI may find their families expect them to take on more burdens in this area than male family members due to gender role expectations. Fulfilling these expectations might interfere with sustaining competitive work outside the home. Alternatively, clinicians can explore the degree to which women with SMI might find pride or meaning in providing domestic labor to their families when they are unable to work outside the home. Providers may also find it helpful to utilize the clinical worksheet located at the end of the chapter, the "Work and Class Worksheet," with women with SMI and others who may benefit.

CONCLUSION

Women with SMI tend to experience their class background as a narrative. This story often includes having lower incomes later in life due to SMI symptoms and stigma. Adding to their financial challenges are gender disparities in employment, wages, and income faced by women in general. Women with SMI confront a number of unique barriers related to work and class compared to their counterparts, including gender and mental illness discrimination, unpaid domestic labor expectations, and risks of homelessness posed by unemployment. These women also carry unique strengths around working, including accessing social support, developing an awareness of sexism and mental illness stigma, and taking on flexible and meaningful work roles that enhance their sense of pride and ability to advocate for themselves and others. Clinicians can help women with SMI to draw from their particular strengths in overcoming challenges to work and financial wellness.

CLINICAL STRATEGIES

- Explore the impact of gender and mental health on women's experience of their class background and work experience. What unique barriers or resources do they encounter as a result of their gender?
- Take a work and class history of women with SMI and explore their current work and financial goals.
- Ask about the multiple marginalized identities that women with SMI may experience in addition to the mental illness identity as they impact class and work. These identities might relate to other disabilities (physical, intellectual, psychiatric), racial-ethnic background, class, education, and homelessness. Investigate how intersectional stigma impacts experiences with work and class.
- Identify any history of discrimination (potentially pertaining to mental illness stigma) in work or education settings that may have posed barriers to academic, professional, and financial achievements.
- Facilitate access to financial resources such as public assistance, housing, and education resources. Case management may be helpful in providing knowledgeable support in this area.
- Find out who has been helping a woman with SMI manage her finances and public assistance, such as a "rep(resentative) payee" or other guardian. Examine and strategize her satisfaction with that relationship. This could occur in individual therapy or a case management meeting, in a family or dyadic session, and/or with the support of legal services. Help the woman to access these resources as needed.
- Support access to supported employment and vocational rehabilitation programs that may be available to help women with SMI to achieve their goals.
- Identify particular strengths and challenges a women with SMI may have as a worker, as well as any particular interests she might have for her future in work, whether paid or unpaid.
- Help her to identify meaningful work that is attainable, perhaps paid or unpaid, that could add purpose and structure to daily life. Discuss the accommodations or flexible arrangements that she might need in order to be successful.

DISCUSSION QUESTIONS

1. Proponents of intersectionality theory argue that a person is not solely defined by one aspect of identity (e.g., gender, race, class). Rather, multiple identities combined uniquely impact experience (e.g., Black woman with SMI who is wealthy). Do you agree with this theory, or do you feel that a woman with an SMI is primarily defined by one

aspect of her identity, such as race, class, or gender? How do you feel intersectionality theory might apply to women with SMI in the working world, perhaps from different sexual orientations, abilities, ages, and racial-ethnic backgrounds? Explain your ideas.

2. How might women with SMI be particularly vulnerable to sexual harassment and discrimination in the workplace? What are some of the potential applications of the #MeToo movement for women with SMI in the workplace?

3. How might class privilege (unearned advantages experienced by people with higher incomes) affect women with SMI in their experiences of education, work, housing, and financial wellness?

ACTIVITIES

1. Money Scripts. Psychologist Brad Klontz, Psy.D., and colleagues (2011) identified problematic money scripts, or beliefs about finances that are linked to economic challenges (particularly the first three scripts in the following list). Identify a person with a mental health problem you are working with or someone in your own life who has discussed problems with financial wellness. Consider administering the Money Script Inventory (Klontz & Britt, 2012, found at https://www.psychologytoday.com/files/attachments/34772/money-beliefs-and-financial-behaviors-development-the-klontz-money-script-inventory-jft-2011.pdf). Now explore the following money scripts from this article as they apply to this person:
   (A) Money avoidance—beliefs that "money is bad, rich people are greedy, and they don't deserve money"
   (B) Money worship—beliefs that "more money will solve all of one's problems, there will never be enough money, and money brings power and happiness"
   (C) Money status—"equate self-worth to net worth and put a premium on buying the newest and best things"
   (D) Money vigilance—beliefs reflecting "themes of frugality, the importance of saving, being discreet about how much money one has or makes, and nervousness about making sure money is saved in case of an emergency."
   How have this person's experiences with family and mental health uniquely affected his or her money scripts? What are some treatment recommendations for uniquely supporting this person in working toward financial wellness?

2. Supported Employment and Vocational Rehabilitation Program. Develop a curriculum outline for a potential supported employment/

vocational rehabilitation program for women with SMI. First, identify several of your goals for the group. Then identify the main topics you would want to address in the group. What potential activities might you include to attain these objectives? Explain how you would support the needs of women with SMI in the workplace, with attention to multiple levels of stigma they may face as women with mental health problems from different demographic backgrounds. In a group, compare and contrast these group curricula. Consider combining into one group to pilot.

Work and Class Worksheet

Class Background/Socioeconomic Status
Childhood:

Adulthood:

Education history:

Work history (paid or unpaid):

Effects of mental health
On school:

On work:

Worker Strengths:	Worker Challenges:
Financial Resources:	Financial Risks:

Work Goals (paid or unpaid):
Two easy steps to work toward goal: 1)
2)

Financial Goals:
Two easy steps to work toward goal: 1)
2)

6

Cultural Factors Among Women with Serious Mental Illness

Race, Gender, Sexuality, and Spirituality

Mental illness is inextricably linked to culture. Culture can impact various aspects of mental illness that one might expect to be unchangeable, including its onset, symptoms, and course (Sam & Morreira, 2012). Culture can also affect a person's understanding and expectations of the illness (Bhugra, 2006; Kleinman, 1988). On the other hand, one's culture can offer vital sources of resilience.

Cultural issues of race, gender, sexuality, and spirituality are clearly interwoven into the lived experiences of women with serious mental illness (SMI). We will examine this complex topic of culture of women with SMI and the intersectional stigma they encounter. Logie and colleagues (2011) defined this concept as the "interdependent and mutually constitutive relationships between marginalized social identities and inequities" (p. 1). The intersectional model can help us to understand the overlapping identities within each individual that contribute to experiences of oppression as well as privilege, or unearned cultural advantages. In several case vignettes of women with SMI, we will explore their experiences with intersectional stigma, and the cultural resources they draw from to overcome it.

RACE, ETHNICITY, AND SMI

Discrimination faced by people with SMI is multilayered and widespread. This type of discrimination often includes both racial discrimination and psychiatric stigma. Corrigan and colleagues (2003) conducted a large study of almost 1,000 participants with SMI in order to understand the different types and incidences of perceived discrimination, including racism. They found the highest rates of perceived discrimination to be reported for mental and physical disability, race, and sexual orientation. There were especially high rates of discrimination reported by participants of color as well as gay and bisexual participants. The participants felt that employers, landlords, and police were the chief perpetrators of discrimination.

Other research on discrimination toward people with SMI has reinforced these findings. In a study of over 200 people with SMI, daily experiences of discrimination were reported by 94% of the sample, with 88% experiencing a history of discrimination in at least one area (Gabbidon et al., 2014). Perceptions of racism had the highest incidence among Black and mixed-race groups. People with two or more oppressed identities also reported very high levels of perceived discrimination, reflecting the aforementioned problem of intersectional stigma. With regard to the perpetration of discrimination, people with SMI ranked their mental health providers and neighbors at the top, followed by law enforcement, employers, and medical care staff and providers. For the participants with SMI, the most frequent reason given for why they felt discrimination occurred was due to their mental illness, followed by their racial-ethnic background, class, and appearance.

This work by Gabbidon and colleagues (2014) seems to suggest that people with SMI perceive multiple aspects of their identities to incur discrimination from a range of personal and professional contacts in their daily lives. There also appears to be a heightened sense of strain for those who belong to both racial and sexual minority groups, and in settings in which they work, live, and receive care. It can be noted that these studies are based on perception, and it is difficult to verify these reports through observational research. Yet the fact that these groups worry on a day-to-day basis about discrimination in so many areas of life speaks to the real consequences of racism and other forms of oppression on psychological well-being (Wise, 2005).

Mental Health Disparities

Differences in the prevalence of SMI among different racial-ethnic groups reveal the effects of racial-ethnic disparities on mental health. According to a review article by Primm and colleagues (2010), the highest prevalence of SMI in the United States was found among American Indians (50% to 54% men, 40% to 46% women), followed by non-Hispanic European Americans (21%), Latino Americans (16%), African Americans (15%), and Asian Americans (9%).

In a 2010 article, Primm and colleagues identified racial-ethnic factors in the recovery process that could interfere with access to care. These obstacles included language and help-seeking barriers, as well as racial disparities in incarceration risks. Low-income immigrant groups could have lower rates of health insurance and be barred by the cost of care. Alternatively, research has found that people of color with SMI have reduced access to mental health services even if they have insurance, partially due to fear of discriminatory care (Thomas & Snowden, 2001). Moreover, some lower-income African Americans may be less likely to pursue outpatient mental health and medical services rather than emergency services. Many American Indians may also be less likely to seek Western mental health services if they live on or near a reservation; rather, they might seek treatment from traditional healers. Racism and fear of discrimination appear to be factors that often lead to higher rates of victimization, abuse, and trauma. Ida (2007) identified a number of findings from the research on racial-ethnic disparities in mental health as they affect recovery from SMI. For one, African Americans are estimated to receive only half the mental health services of White Americans. Native Americans tend to have high rates of alcohol-related mortality, as well as suicide and homicide rates. LGBT populations also have elevated suicide and homicide rates. Many of these disparities are likely to result from discrimination and minority stress, as well as cross-generational effects of oppression on mental health among populations of color.

Cultural research on people with SMI has led to the identification of some cultural trends across groups. For example, in an article on Chinese people with SMI, Chen and Mak (2008) suggested that collectivist cultural values in Asian groups might be linked to internal attributions of mental health problems, which can lead to high levels of stigma toward mental illness. In this study and others (see Okazaki, 2000), researchers have identified trends in the research that suggest relatively low rates of treatment utilization among East Asian individuals who are born in the United States or are more recent immigrants. Furthermore, the results of older studies have shown that Asian Americans may encounter treatment bias and higher incidences of psychotic disorder diagnoses than their White counterparts (Akutsu, Snowden, & Organista, 1996; Flaskerud & Hu, 1992).

With regard to Latino mental health, the findings of one study suggest that it is common for Latino Americans with SMI to experience co-occurring mood, anxiety, and substance use disorders (Sánchez et al., 2017). Another study found that Latinos also had greater post-traumatic stress disorder (PTSD) symptoms compared to African Americans and White Americans with SMI (O'Hare, Shen, & Sherrer, 2017). Trauma history has also been associated with a greater risk for suicidality among Latino clients with SMI compared to African Americans and White Americans (O'Hare, Shen, & Sherrer, 2016). Other research on Latinos with SMI has found that the incidence of psychiatric disorders is lower for Latinos than non-Latino Whites (Alegría et al., 2008). These authors explored the immigrant paradox—the idea that more recent immigrants have fewer psychiatric disorders and other health issues than more established immigrants in the United States. This concept was demonstrated in their findings that U.S.-born Latinos had more problems with mental health than non–U.S-born Latinos.

Several studies have found a number of health disparities for people with SMI who are African American. These inequities likely tend to result from cross-generational effects of slavery on economic, sociocultural, and mental health outcomes (DeGruy, 2005). For example, in a study by Lo and Cheng (2014), African American participants had an increased risk of developing SMI during times of economic challenge in comparison to their White counterparts. Those authors cited research on the social disadvantages of minority stress, including barriers to health care access. They identified the effects of racism on the development of SMI, symptom severity, and barriers to treatment. Lo and Cheng also found an increase in unemployment for people with SMI, particularly for African

Americans compared to White Americans during a recession, even when demographic factors were controlled for.

In a study of African Americans with SMI, the participants had lower than average improvements in functioning, activation, and other symptoms and were less likely return to work in the year after a hospitalization (Eack & Newhill, 2012). These racial disparities were present even after adjusting for sociodemographic variables such as gender, socioeconomic status, and diagnosis. Problems with treatment access and quality were likely to be responsible for these differences.

The disenfranchisement of African Americans with SMI in the U.S. mental health system is manifold (Eack & Newhill, 2012). African Americans are more likely to receive medications at higher doses and injection medications than their White counterparts. They are more likely to receive older antipsychotics with more side effects, even though African Americans metabolize medications in a way that require need lower-than-typical dosages. They are more likely to be misdiagnosed with psychotic disorders rather than affective disorders. And they are more likely to be involuntarily hospitalized, often with police force due to perceptions of dangerousness. The mental health experiences of many African Americans with SMI reveal the effects of racial oppression on the development, course, and treatment of people with SMI.

Explanatory Models

A key cultural difference across racial-ethnic groups with SMI has to do with explanatory models. Explanatory models are the way we understand the root cause of an illness and make meaning of it (Kleinman, 1988). Carpenter-Song and colleagues (2010) conducted a study to explore these differences in cultural explanations of SMI across racial-ethnic groups. According to this study, the cultural explanatory models of illness among many African Americans tend to be non-biomedical. Some African Americans might view SMI as a private matter, feel critical of medications, and see Western medical approaches to SMI as impersonal or narrow in focus. Many African Americans might also feel a cultural mistrust toward mental health providers due to a history of mistreatment (Carpenter-Song et al., 2010; Nickerson, Helms, & Terrell, 1994).

Another study found the African American participants tended to express explanatory models of SMI as more character-based, or resulting from sociocultural factors (Alverson et al., 2007). These participants tended to prefer talk therapy, which was seen as a more personal intervention. Daily, concrete problems with housing, food, transportation, unemployment, poverty, and racial discrimination were often viewed as just as important as the SMI. Other studies also suggest that many African Americans with SMI may find it difficult to discern whether they are experiencing stigma toward their race or their mental illness given the often masked nature of bias (Armour, Bradshaw, & Roseborough, 2009).

While Latino Americans are a particularly diverse group spanning many different nationalities, some commonalities in explanatory models have emerged.

This cultural explanatory model tends to highlight the physical nature of SMI, but not from a biomedical framework (Carpenter-Song et al., 2010). This view can reduce the stigma associated with mental health problems, although Western diagnostic labels are often highly associated with stigma, and thus avoided. Mental and medical health providers may be seen by some Latinos as intermediaries for obtaining medication or other medical interventions. They may also have mixed feelings about the utility of these treatments.

One study found that Puerto Rican participants tended to avoid diagnostic labels and see them as stigmatizing or incongruent with cultural views of SMI (Alverson et al., 2007). SMI was more likely to be seen as an emotional problem or an understandable reaction to disrespect. Herbal treatments (*botánicos remédicos*) and *herbalistas* might be used as part of their care. Similar to the findings of Carpenter-Song and colleagues (2010), talk therapy was viewed as a process of "just going through the motions" to acquire medication or disability paperwork (Alverson et al., 2007).

Alverson and colleagues (2007) also examined the cultural explanatory models of White Americans with SMI, a group whose perspective we often take for granted as part of the compulsory normalization of the dominant culture. White American participants clearly had their own unique cultural views of SMI, viewing the illness as permanent and disabling. The SMI was often understood as originating within the individual. Thus, White Americans with SMI appear to be prone to becoming isolated, and the responsibility for pursuing treatment is often seen as lying within the individual. They found that White Americans often have biomedical and disease-oriented explanations for the cause of SMI, emphasizing the role of medication in treatment and preventing hospitalizations. At best, this viewpoint could encourage adherence to effective treatments, but at worst, it could promote a sick role identity, as well as passivity to achieving recovery.

These studies indicate the various mental health disparities across racial-ethnic lines that impact the development and treatment of SMI. However, there are several caveats to remember in interpreting these results. For one, race is a social construct, and there is more biological diversity within racial-ethnic groups than between them. However, the effects of racism have real implications for medical and mental health, as shown by the aforementioned literature. Much of the research on racial-ethnic groups looks at averages across groups and can risk generalizations and stereotypes. All of this means that the mental health findings we have described in this section contain important information about cultural trends but can overlook within-group differences, and should therefore be interpreted with caution.

Another caveat is with regard to racial-ethnic disparities. When we examine problems within a culture, we must balance this perspective with an understanding of the associated sources of cultural resilience and strength. Just one of these potential sources of cultural resilience has to do with an empowering engagement with spiritual and religious practices and groups. Hence, we will focus on these important spiritual facilitators to recovery in a later section. Before that, we will explore another marginalized group with SMI, people who are LGBT.

LGBT INDIVIDUALS WITH SMI

Like other marginalized groups, LGBT groups face societal stigma that can lead to an increased risk of mental health problems and intersectional stigma. LGBT-related stigma has been linked to increased incidences of mental disorders, suicidality, and victimization (Kidd et al., 2011; Mays & Cochran, 2001; Mustanski, Garofalo, & Emerson, 2010). LGBT individuals who encounter stigma may come to internalize the stigma, directing prejudice inward (Hellman & Klein, 2004). Internalized stigma, also known as self-stigma, may worsen attempts at socialization and functioning and interfere with quality of life, contributing to a negative sense of self (Hellman & Klein, 2004; Kidd et al., 2011). Furthermore, maladaptive coping strategies (e.g., substance use, eating disorders, self-harm) might be used to deal with internalized stigma and prejudice, as captured in the "minority stress model" (Meyer, 2003).

One study found that reports of discrimination among individuals with mental illness were highest among LGBT individuals (Corrigan et al., 2003). Intersectional stigma among LGBT individuals with mental illness may inhibit disclosure of mental health problems, interfering with access to rehabilitation services that promote recovery (Cook, 2000). Intersectional stigma can also contribute to financial and social difficulties for LGBT people with SMI. Barriers to employment, insurance, family financial support, and partner benefits in many states create financial stress, worsening mental health (Hellman & Klein, 2004).

Furthermore, individuals with SMI may become alienated from the rest of the LGBT community, and vice versa, reducing the social support needed to facilitate acceptance of mental illness (Hellman & Klein, 2004). People with SMI often rely on family members for practical and emotional support, increasing stress for LGBT individuals who have been rejected by family members (Lucksted, 2004). LGBT individuals with mental illness also report barriers to dating and finding a life partner due to hospitalizations in early adulthood (Barber, 2009). Intersectional stigma encountered by LGBT individuals with mental illness can interfere with relationship building and social functioning, increasing isolation (Kidd et al., 2011).

LGBT individuals with mental illness also report reduced treatment satisfaction and high rates of discrimination within mental health settings (Hellman, Sudderth, & Avery, 2002; Kidd et al., 2011). Bias on the part of clinicians can interfere with LGBT clients' acceptance, trust, and participation in outpatient, inpatient, and emergency mental health services (Hellman et al., 2010; Ziguras et al., 2003). LGBT people are sometimes desexualized and dehumanized in treatment settings (Lucksted, 2004) or, conversely, hypersexualized for their gender or sexual identities. There may be silence around LGBT identity in the mental health system due to a history of mistreatment, as well as a lack of knowledge and training among providers. Staff might also condone transphobia or homophobia through ignoring or not acting on it, requiring LGBT individuals to be hypervigilant about stigma in the mental health system.

Transgender and gender-diverse people with SMI may face other challenges in mental health settings. They often feel burdened to educate their health care providers, who are often untrained in this area, taking them out of the patient role and putting them into the educator role (Lucksted, 2004; Mizock & Lundquist, 2016). While at times this role may be empowering for the client, it can also take attention away from the focus needed on one's own treatment. Staff may evaluate the wellness of transgender individuals based on their identification with their birth gender (Lucksted, 2004). Transgender individuals also report alienation by LGB peers in particular and may be hesitant to enroll in inpatient treatment or participate in groups for fear of peer ostracization (Hellman & Klein, 2004; Hellman et al., 2010).

Transgender people face increased risk of mental health problems compared to their cisgender and LGB counterparts. According to another study, 20% to 50% of trans-feminine people experience a major mental illness and 26% to 62% experience a history of substance abuse (Nutbrock et al., 2010). Rates of eating disorders and body image disturbances, as well as anxiety and depressive disorders, are also high compared to the general population (Mizock, 2017). The lifetime prevalence of attempted suicide among transgender individuals has been estimated at an alarming rate of 32% (Clements-Nolle et al., 2006). These rates of psychiatric distress and mental illness have been largely attributed to societal stigma, including factors such as peer bullying, family rejection, and abuse history (Leibowitz & Telingator, 2012).

The controversial diagnosis of Gender Dysphoria in the fifth edition of the American Psychiatric Association's *Diagnostic and Statistical Manual of Mental Disorders* ([DSM-5], 2013), formerly Gender Identity Disorder (DSM-IV-TR, 2000), continues to label many trans people as having a mental disorder. The DSM-5 diagnosis of Gender Dysphoria includes persistent discomfort with one's biological sex, significant distress, and/or impairment in functioning. While including Gender Dysphoria in the DSM may support insurance reimbursement for gender-related care, it can be argued that the inclusion of this diagnosis continues to stigmatize transgender individuals by naming this identity as a mental illness altogether, harkening back to the days when homosexuality was also a diagnosis in the DSM.

SPIRITUALITY AND SMI

A key factor that can help overcome stigma and other challenges associated with SMI is a positive connection to religion and spirituality. Positive religious and spiritual beliefs and family support have been identified as key cultural protective factors in the development of SMI (Primm et al., 2010). Some denominational programs have even been developed to support and minister to people with mental health concerns, as listed on the National Alliance on Mental Illness (NAMI)'s FaithNet website (https://www.nami.org/faithnet).

Spirituality and religion appear to have assorted mental health and physical benefits. Previous research has found positive effects of religious involvement (i.e., service attendance and religious practices) for mental health, including reduced anxiety, depression, alcohol and substance use and greater self-esteem, motivation, and quality of life (see Gupta & Gupta, 2014). There also appear to be benefits of religion for physical well-being, recovery from illness, and positive health behaviors. Some specific illnesses have been found to be less common in religious individuals, including hypertension, physical disability, stroke, and cancer.

One study of religious and spiritual practices among Indian men and women shed light on the benefits of positive practices and beliefs on mental health. Gupta and Gupta (2014) found that the men and women who participated the most in religious and spiritual practices had the highest scores of religious commitment, life satisfaction, optimism, and meaning in life, with lower scores on stress and anxiety. Women had higher levels of religious commitment than men. Women's religious commitment was associated with more optimism and life satisfaction and lower levels of stress and anxiety.

In fact, recovery from SMI has been presented as a religious process in itself (Lukoff, 2007). Recovery has been construed as a journey involving spiritual questions about one's relationship to God and reasons for the illness. According to several studies, 30% to 90% of people have reported spirituality and religion to be one of the most important parts of recovery from mental illnesses (Fallot, 2007). Many people report an increase of faith after a psychotic episode, as they may seek spiritual guidance to deal with the symptoms of the illness (Fallot, 2008; Lukoff, 2007; Miller & McCormack, 2006). People have often reported a benefit from knowing they can still have authentic connections to God despite a diagnosis of SMI (Lukoff, 2007). Deegan (2011) put forth the somewhat controversial notion that psychotic thoughts may even help to access spirituality for many people with SMI.

Fallot (2008) provided a helpful guide to dealing with these potential risks and benefits for individuals with SMI in therapy interventions:

1. There may be benefits associated with inclusion. Some religious communities are inclusive and welcoming of individuals with SMI, offering acceptance and support. However, other religious and spiritual communities may reject individuals with SMI, may be homophobic, or may discourage the use of psychiatric medication and traditional medical supports.
2. Individuals with SMI may feel empowered as someone who is valued by the divine within their religious involvement. On the other hand, they may feel devalued within a religion if they are seen as someone who is being punished with a mental illness for past sins.
3. Religion could offer coping strategies for expression and relief, including prayer, meditation, and other behavioral rituals that add structure or

self-expression to the day. In contrast, the expected religious rituals might contribute to a sense of rigidity and compulsivity.

4. Religion could offer a sense of autonomy through liberation from a strict reliance on traditional psychiatric care (Fallot, 2008). However, some religious beliefs might overemphasize external control without championing an internal capacity to alter one's life circumstances.

5. Religion could offer hope as it can boost energy and calmness, enthusiasm, joy, and motivation through meditative practices of prayer and connection. Alternatively, religion could lead to increased feelings of despair by reinforcing a sense of sinfulness, guilt, and hopelessness in reaching salvation.

Some research on religion and SMI has explored the role of religious delusions in psychosis. The literature in mental illness and religiosity has often focused on the association of demonic, satanic delusions with violent behaviors (Mohr & Huguelet, 2006). While this is important to address, over-focusing on this topic risks negative stereotypes of religious beliefs for people with SMI. A minority of people with SMI tends to hold these types of delusions, and they are generally not acted on (Miller & McCormack, 2006).

It is also imperative to differentiate a mystical, spiritual, or transcendental experience from a delusion. Some spiritual experiences are culturally congruent rather than reflective of psychopathology (Mohr & Huguelet, 2006). A transcendental spiritual experience may be a positive one, differing from a psychotic delusion in that the former is typically followed by a return to reality and is often considered acceptable within the individual's religion. People with SMI might be able to recover from the acute distress of a delusion and draw from positive religious resources with support and without confrontation of the delusion (Fallot, 2008).

Cultural Differences in Religious and Spiritual Practices Among People with SMI

Religious or spiritual beliefs that enable positive coping behaviors and social support have been associated with resilience and reduced levels of mental illness among people with SMI who are racial, gender, and sexual minorities (Golub et al., 2010; Lo, Cheng, & Howell, 2014). This is in addition to other resilience factors for marginalized groups, like identity pride, peer support, and activism (Mizock, 2017). Religious practices may have different implications for mental health depending on one's specific racial-ethnic identity. For example, studies of the spiritual practices of African Americans have found that many individuals in this group may be more likely to use prayer, the Bible, church attendance, and the church community as coping strategies for dealing with mental health stressors (Abernethy et al., 2006). A qualitative study with religious African Americans with SMI identified themes with regard to a belief and sense in unity with God

(Armour et al., 2009). The participants found solace in traditional African spiritual beliefs. The participants found involvement in church to be helpful in offering a sense of community interdependence in overcoming racial oppression.

With regard to Latino cultures, Cervantes (2010) highlighted the impact of colonization of indigenous Latin American forms of religion and spirituality. Many original practices were eradicated by Europeans and replaced with Western traditions, creating a mix of indigenous and Christian and Catholic religions. Contemporary religious practices are often characterized by worship of deities and shrines, devotional offerings, prayer, and pilgrimages. Mestizo spirituality among Mexican and Mexican American groups often reflects religious values in diversity and connectedness to the social and physical environment. They also often honor life stories and the memories of deceased loved ones.

Again, there is also a large degree of diversity across tribal groups within Native American cultures (American Psychiatric Association, 2010; LaFromboise, Trimble, & Mohatt, 1990). Many Native American groups do not segment spirituality from the rest of daily life, but rather provide a spiritual infusion throughout daily life and culture. Some tribal groups initially viewed psychotic-like states as having a spiritual value to the culture. However, the influence of Western values has led many Native American groups to come to see mental illness as more stigmatizing (Dakota-Lakota-Nakota Human Rights Advocacy Coalition, 2002). European colonization also brought Christianity to the current religious practice of many members of Native American groups and other global cultures (LaFromboise et al., 1990). It should also be noted that traditional American Indian healing systems take a holistic approach to treating the mind, body, and spirit, integrating a sense of connection to one's cultural homeland (American Psychiatric Association, 2010).

Hanna and Green (2004) examined the multicultural counseling implications of three Asian religions—Hinduism, Buddhism, and Islam. They indicated that practices of Hinduism and Buddhism may involve meditation techniques that reduce anxiety and distress from psychotic symptoms. This might include the Shvetashvatara Upanishad in the Hindu religion or walking meditation and mindfulness exercises in Buddhist meditation. In the case of Islamic individuals with SMI, there may be spiritual values of benevolence, personal development, and forgiveness that can be of focus in therapy. Clearly, there are many more religious practices in Asian groups and other cultures that could offer mental health benefits. More information can be sought in other readings (see, e.g., Koenig, 1998; Tewari & Alvarez, 2009).

Religion and spirituality are also sources of resilience for some LGBT individuals (Merryman & Mizock, 2016), including those with SMI. Religious and spiritually based coping appear to be a key link in the reduction of mental health symptoms for LGBT people, particularly when it promotes social support. Though many places of worship have historically rejected LGBT individuals, many religious communities are LGBT affirming, providing helpful spiritual teachings and a space for connection. A growing number of LGBT individuals belong to affirmative congregations and even become religious leaders in these institutions, seeking spiritual answers for the challenges they face in their communities and finding a greater sense of purpose and meaning.

Women's Spirituality

Women-centered religions may also offer unique resources for coping with mental health challenges to women with SMI. Women-centered religions differ from male-centered ones in a number of ways. For example, feminine-focused spiritual practices are often non-hierarchical in their structure, with circular movement instead of being progressive and linear (Briggs & Dixon, 2013; Lauver, 2000). This is in contrast to traditional religious orders that place God in the most powerful role, followed by men, women, and animals. Matriarchal religions often include feminine characterizations of the divine (Briggs & Dixon, 2013; Lauver, 2000). Inclusive language is also used to refer to the divine: Instead of Father, Son, and the Holy Ghost, gender-neutral terms may be used such as the Creator, Redeemer, or Sustainer. Alternatively, feminine terms for divinity may be used, like "Goddess" (Lauver, 2000). Feminist spirituality emphasizes a greater power that promotes love, justice, and equity (Briggs & Dixon, 2013). There is a focus on ethnic diversity and an emphasis on empowerment and deconstructing traditional, patriarchal religious beliefs and practices (Lauver, 2000).

Lauver (2000) detailed some of the common spiritual practices in women-centered religions, such as dancing, music, cooking, placing flowers on graves, burning symbolic items to let them go, thematic readings in groups, reflective discussion, meditation, singing, or other exercises. There may be celebrations to mark developmental milestones for women, such as menstruation, divorce, coming out, or recovery from addiction.

Another intersection of gender and race for women with SMI is the womanist spiritual tradition. This tradition was born in African American women's critique of the White history of feminism, which has often been non-inclusive or exploitative of women of color (Heath, 2006). In contrast, womanist spirituality is historically situated in African tradition and ancestry. Heath (2006) identified womanist spirituality as a valuable resource for mental health recovery of women of color with SMI. She described womanism as a form of social justice and political protest in the face of oppression and violence—a "psychological resistance strategy" where spirituality can enhance health, healing, and coping for Black women.

As seen in this literature, race and ethnicity as well as sexuality, religion, and spirituality are cultural factors that hold implications for the experiences of women with SMI. The next section will include several case narratives from our research that illuminate issues of race, ethnicity, gender, and spiritual-religious practice as they impact the experiences of women with SMI. The case narratives will explore each individual's cultural identity, mental health, spirituality, and religion. Applications to clinical work will be presented based on these stories in order to inform the mental health support of other women with SMI from diverse racial-ethnic and spiritual-religious backgrounds.

CASE NARRATIVES

Case 1: Raya

"Raya" is a Black and Asian American, bisexual, Pagan woman in her 40s. She identifies as polyamorous and pansexual. She has a history of severe depression and other mental health challenges, as well as physical disabilities, including a chronic pain condition, fibromyalgia. Raya understands her complex trauma history of sexual and emotional abuse throughout her youth as having impacted her mental and physical health. She grew up in an educated, middle-class family. However, she lost her parents and survived numerous physical and sexual traumas at an early age. Substance abuse, homelessness, and chronic poverty followed her into adulthood, worsened by the mental health and physical challenges that interfered with her ability to work.

Raya discussed the intersectional stigma she encounters with regard to sexism, racism, and mental illness stigma:

Being a woman in this culture, you get mistreated walking down the street. You know it's gotten really ridiculous, the level of sexism in this country after 9/11. I think our country went back to the 1950s . . . in 2001. Being Black, I've had my own issues . . . A lot of people don't even know me. And by the time someone knows me, they know that I have a mental illness. They know that I have health issues, and they know that I have an anxiety disorder . . . I've gotten catcalls and . . . I've gotten my fair share of shit.

Raya identified the different levels on which she encountered discrimination depending on what aspect of her selfhood was visible. While race and gender were visible identities that incurred marginalization, her psychiatric and health conditions might be less visible to others.

Raya spoke to her challenging experiences with race as someone with mixed racial heritage:

I'd say being half Black and half Indian is really interesting, because there's such a taboo against Indian guys sleeping with anyone who's not Indian that I've never felt part of the Indian community . . . My uncle basically ostracized my dad. And when we would go into Indian places, I noticed the way my dad got treated for having us, and it wasn't good . . . I don't know that many Indian people. And being Black, it's been interesting. But it's like, you're Black but you're not Black. So, it's more of a question of racial identity still in this country.

Raya's experience as someone of mixed race in American culture led her to feel not fully accepted in either community. At times, she became a target of internalized and intergroup racism. This struggle with belonging added to the pain of racism, mental illness stigma, classism, and sexism in her experience of intersectional stigma.

Gender was another area in which Raya was able to pinpoint experiences of discrimination. When asked about particular mistreatment women with SMI might experience in mental health services, she described some of her observations of gender issues in inpatient psychiatric units:

> I think that guys are allowed to get away with being a lot more out of control and a little bit more violent than women are. . . . The guys—they have a tendency to yell and scream and aren't called on it. But if a woman would yell and scream, she would be called on it in a second . . . I think it's unfair. And I think it's bullshit. And it really bothers me that . . . sometimes it feels like any time a woman opens her mouth that somebody is looking to silence her.

One of the areas of her life that brings her meaning in dealing with her struggles is her identification with non-Christian religions. She is connected to the West African traditional religion of Vodun (often referred to as Voodoo, the somewhat Christianized form), and the Ordo Templi Orientis (OTO) popularized by the English author and occultist Aleister Crowley. She described the role of religion in her life:

> I'm Pagan. My great-grandma was Vodun from New Orleans. We were sort of related to Marie Laveau in a weird way that my great-grandma could have explained if she was alive. But we come from Vodun ancestry on their side and they were Catholic. And my dad was Hindu until the partition of India until he was about 15 years old. When he got to England, he joined Aleister Crowley's magical group, the OTO. So I'm my own really weird version of an eclectic Pagan.

Though religion and spirituality have been positive sources of resilience, Raya has faced health and financial barriers to participating in and claiming these religions:

> I don't identify a lot with the actual Order anymore because I grew up in it, and I saw the good side as well as the bad side of my religion . . . Vodun is its own world. . . . I do individual spell work stuff but . . . I don't consider myself part of a Vodun community. You would have to make a real commitment to a real Vodun community. And that's a lot of energy that I don't have because I have fibromyalgia. I can't do the ritual commitment of that.

Though her physical and psychiatric disabilities might interfere with her participation in her religion, she finds ways to keep her practice going:

> I would say I do a lot of solitary work. I go to the occasional ritual thrown by the OTO when I need to, like if there are people I want to actually see. Like

last year I went to this great big huge art thing for my birthday, which was my birthday gift to myself. I actually volunteered for it, and it was amazing.

Raya's story highlights the complex intersecting identities of women with SMI with regard to race, gender, class, and disability. Her awareness of stigma in one area of her identity enhanced her awareness of oppression in her other identities. Her diverse cultural identities were also inclusive of multiple religious and spiritual practices—all of which she wove together to foment her recovery and well-being.

Case 2: Kris

"Kris" is a White American person in their thirties who was raised Catholic. Because Kris identifies as genderqueer (people who do not align with binary notions of gender and identify with neither, both, or a combination of male and female genders), the pronouns "they" and "their" will be used in this vignette, a standard practice with nonbinary people. Kris currently identifies as asexual but has a history of identifying as lesbian. With regard to gender, Kris identifies as both a woman and as genderqueer. Kris discussed their gender affirmation process and challenges posed by the SMI:

When I first realized it, I think it was strongest. Now it's just something that I sort of know and sit with. And I just say to myself, "You know, there will be a time when this will be addressed. I'm not giving up on it." . . . Unfortunately this year I've been too symptomatic with my post-traumatic stress to focus on that.

With regard to another important aspect of identity, race, Kris responded:

I'm not really sure. I know my grandmother on my mother's side was 100% Italian. My mother's biological father, I believe, was English, maybe Irish? Or French? And then I don't know about my dad's side. I think given some of the names, like genealogy-wise, and where I grew up in upstate New York, I think they might be Dutch, or something like that.

Kris's difficulty identifying their ethnic background is not uncommon for many White Americans in the United States. The social construction of whiteness in America has brought with it a number of unearned societal advantages afforded to those with racial privilege (Cushman, 1995). Conversely, White identification has brought with it this loss of one's cultural history and selfhood.

Kris has a history of PTSD and severe depression with psychotic features. Like Raya, Kris's SMI appears to have been triggered by a number of emotional, physical, and sexual traumas that Kris has survived as well as other hardships. Kris grew up in rural poverty. The family members needed to boil water to take baths. They ate much of their food from their garden, and Kris's father and grandfather hunted and ice fished for sustenance. Kris's parents divorced when Kris was a child due to their father's alcoholism and violence. Kris moved with their mother to an East Coast city where she worked as an administrative assistant.

Kris escaped the abuse of their father, their stepfather, and later their own abusive partner. After fleeing this partner, Kris was hospitalized in an inpatient program. Adding insult to injury, Kris was pursued sexually by a counselor at this facility. Kris developed the courage to report the counselor's behavior. It took some convincing of the staff of the legitimacy of their complaints, but the counselor was eventually fired from the mental health center. Kris perceived sexism in this episode of their mental health treatment, intersecting with stigma toward their mental illness:

> I feel that because I am a woman who had a restraining order, with real domestic violence, probably the worst domestic violence that I've ever encountered personally to my own self, that because I had a mental illness that I was not believed by either my doctor, the establishment, [or] my social worker . . . And I think if I didn't have a mental illness, or if it was a different situation, if it wasn't a mental hospital, and I was just walking in off the street to get resources, and they didn't know I had X diagnosis, and didn't know I was in X hospital, then I would have been treated differently. I feel that strongly.

Kris also experienced sexism and misogyny in their family. Kris linked negative feelings toward their gender experiences to a complex history of trauma, as well as gender socialization by their mother:

> My period is very triggering to me. I know it has to do with my PTSD, but it's like, the first thing I think of is that it's gross, it's dirty, it's this, that, and the other. All negative. Which was what my mother was telling me, you know? . . . When I wanted to use tampons to help me, she wouldn't buy them for me. And when I bought them, I was a slut. So it's not that people love their periods. But I grew up really thinking I was just a mess. Just dirty and shameful. [That] it was something I should hide. She wouldn't even say it's my "period." It was "the thing." I couldn't say, "I need pads," or she would say, "Do you need 'those things'?" You know? It was very shameful and . . . kept behind [closed doors], secretive. And now it's like, I'm glad I don't have it. And I think in part it has a lot to do with [those experiences].

Kris discussed how their mother perpetuated a societal obsession with female appearance that contributed negatively to their mental health experiences from a young age:

> My mom was very preoccupied with the changes in my body. Like when I was 12. I mean, I'd overhear her talking to her friends. And she'd even talk to me about how small my breasts were, and the ideal is for them to be really

big. And you know, how my butt was curving, and that was going to attract
boys. And I was going to get myself in so-called trouble. All this stuff, you
know? So when I was raped . . . I finally got enough courage to tell my mom.
And the first thing she said was, "What were you wearing?" And I was like,
"What does that matter?"

Kris's mother likely projected her own internalized misogyny from the dominant
culture onto her child. Some mothers might police their daughter's appearance
as an unconscious form of protection, unwittingly teaching them to conform to
gender norms in order to lessen the backlash they might face in the broader culture (Taylor, Whittier, & Rapp, 2009). This gender policing can become severe and
rise to the level of emotional abuse, as in Kris's experience.

Kris was aware how internalizing this sexism from their upbringing could have
contributed to their development of SMI:

[What] I was brought up thinking was that you are supposed to find a
man who loves you and take[s] care of you and so on. I know differently
now . . . I also had an eating disorder, because I thought the skinnier I was,
which was such a focus, the more I'd be loved. I grew my hair out. I thought
the longer my hair was, the more I'd be loved. I mean it was outrageous. It
just became . . . it was all about striving to get the love that I deserved all
along, and didn't get, and thought I would get by being these things that my
mom valued, which were superficial, really.

Though Kris often felt oppressed by the pressure to conform to feminine ideals,
they also found identifying with femininity as empowering at times:

When I'm working really hard on something that I need to fight my way
through or get past, I think of myself as a female warrior. You know, like
with a shield and armor and just really strong and empowered. I think about
women, and they have the ability to give birth and have life, and give birth
to life. And that to me is like an abundance of, I want to say magical, but it's
just like powerful. It's symbolic of giving life and putting life into the world.
I see that as strength. I see single moms working hard to protect their children and putting their children first. And that's not something I had. And
I see people that do that and that to me is admirable in and of itself. But I feel
almost a reverence towards it because it was something that never happened
in my life. So I find women to be very strong.

Kris's gender identification wasn't the only identity that shifted over time. Kris
also described changes in their spiritual and religious practice:

I was brought up Catholic, like very strict Catholic. And over the years I'd
say that I'm not in any one religion. I like the Unitarian Universalist Church
because it takes from all sorts of spiritual leaders and poets and authors and

scientists and many cultures. So that's my favorite church to go to. I like a combination of Buddhism and Paganism. I guess that's where I'm at. I'm like more of a free spirit than someone who wants to be in an organized religion.

Kris discussed a spiritual connection to nature and creativity as central to their recovery from SMI:

It's such a huge stress and anxiety reliever. Just being in nature. Just observing and being submerged in nature or being near the ocean. I am a writer, and I am an artist, so I'm observing it with all my senses. And then I'm also thinking of ways to put it on paper, either in words or with paint. So I'm constantly thinking about all these different things. And I could be at the wharf in the middle of the city but I feel like I'm in this respite. And I'm not anxious. I'm not stressed. I'm not thinking about, worrying about the future. Or going into my past. It brings me right to the present, but it's like I'm awe-inspired . . . I just am. I feel blessed for all that is around me . . . I had a couple different teachers that were talking about Buddhism so I started reading Thích Nhất Hạnh and . . . Eckhart Tolle. About mindfulness and being in the now. And then when I'm in nature, knowing that I am submerged in life.

Like Raya, Kris's story reflects intersectional stigma for people with SMI who face misogyny. Their narrative also highlights the empowerment offered in creative connections to gender and spirituality. An awareness of how intersectional stigma has operated in Kris's life has empowered them to de-internalize oppression.

UNDERSTANDING CULTURAL AND SPIRITUAL FACTORS FOR WOMEN WITH SMI

These case narratives bring to life the research on cultural oppression, highlighting the challenges associated with race, gender, and sexuality for women with SMI, as well as some of the potential resources offered by cultural and spiritual practices. Raya's case illuminates some of the challenges of mixed-race identity as well, and the feeling of being in a liminal identity status, not fully accepted by either racial-ethnic community. However, her diverse background provided her access to a variety of religious and spiritual practices, and she was able to create some of her own blended rituals. Raya and Kris were both aware of how female gender identification had led them to experience hardships and mistreatment by providers, peers, and family members into whom they had put their trust. Their experiences of sexism also appeared to help them to have an awareness of how oppression operated in other aspects of their life, such as in the experience of race, gender, and/or poverty. Notably, they were both survivors of major sexual and physical traumas, a source of oppression often experienced by women with SMI, and a key risk factor in the development of an SMI. Positive religious and spiritual practices afforded them a sense of peace and well-being in the face of mental health challenges.

This chapter highlighted the need for future research in a number of clinical areas, many of which have been noted in the extant literature. For one, researchers need to investigate the double stigma of race and mental illness (Gabbidon et al., 2014). More research on interventions can evaluate the effect of culture on illness; these findings could help providers develop community interventions (Primm et al., 2010). Culturally sensitive treatment for SMI could enhance treatment utilization and satisfaction (Alverson et al., 2007). We also need to better understand the effects of spiritual and religious practices and variations across racial-ethnic groups of women with SMI. Research on race and SMI tends to focus on intervention outcomes, but there is also a need for more research that captures subjective recovery experiences (Armour et al., 2009), as in this chapter. In terms of research and clinical practice, issues of racism, sexism, colonization, homophobia, and poverty must be seen as important factors in the recovery process (Ida, 2007).

APPLICATIONS TO CLINICAL WORK

A number of specific applications to clinical work can emerge from this chapter. For one, clinicians need to address the intersectional stigma of sexism, racism, homophobia, transphobia, poverty, and mental illness. People with SMI from underserved communities have often testified to their mistreatment in mental health settings, or the invisibility of their diverse identities in treatment.

Clinicians can shine a light on the multicultural backgrounds of women with SMI. They can inquire about women's racial-ethnic, sexual, and gender identifications, as well as their history and connection to these identities. Providers can inquire about any experiences with discrimination and prejudice they may have encountered as well as experiences of privilege or unearned societal advantages. They can also learn about how experiences with racial, gender, and sexual oppression might intersect with mental illness stigma. Providers might reference the aforementioned literature on racial-ethnic disparities in mental health care in order to understand a client; however, they should proceed with caution given the great variation within each racial-ethnic group. It is also important to explore the explanatory models that each woman with SMI might have in understanding the cause of, nature of, course of, and treatment for her condition within her particular cultural framework.

LGBT people with SMI are another underserved group in mental health treatment. LGBT individuals have expressed feeling that their sexual and gender-diverse identities are invisible or marginalized in treatment settings. Again, providers should inquire as to the way in which women with SMI might identify their sexual and gender identities and must avoid making assumptions based on appearance. Thus, queer women with SMI should be screened for risk of suicidality given the minority stress faced by this group; providers should emphasize protective factors such as community connectedness and identity pride.

With regard to religion and spirituality, mental health interventions can be culturally adapted to fit the religious and spiritual practices and beliefs of a particular group (Abernethy, Houston, Mimms, & Boyd-Franklin, 2006). Some ways of invoking positive connections to spirituality are listed in the following Clinical Strategies section, including spiritual genograms, prayer, meditation, and various means of creative expression of spirituality. That section also lists more information on how to explore the specific benefits and risks women with SMI might face in their religious affiliation. Providers may also find it helpful to utilize the clinical worksheet located at the end of the chapter, the "Cultural Strengths and Stigma Worksheet," with women with SMI and others who may benefit.

CONCLUSION

This chapter has demonstrated the effects of intersectional stigma on the lives of women with SMI—the overlapping, multiple levels of oppression and privilege faced by women with SMI, particularly with regard to racism, mental illness stigma, and misogyny. It is evident that these women embody strengths, resilience, and empowerment in overcoming the challenges of intersectional stigma and connecting to positive cultural and spiritual resources. A major takeaway of this chapter is that culturally responsive care for women with SMI involves treatment that is gender-sensitive, LGBT-affirmative, anti-racist, anti-classist, and social justice-oriented.

CLINICAL STRATEGIES

- Ask women with SMI how they identify their race, ethnicity, sexuality, gender, and religion.
- Explore any experiences with oppression, privilege, and/or resilience within each of these cultural backgrounds.
- Take a cross-generational family history of these different cultural backgrounds and narratives for the woman with SMI. This process could be conducted using cultural genograms (see Hardy & Lazloffy, 1995). Identify mental health challenges, stigma, and other relevant patterns in the woman's family trajectories.
- Help the woman to identify the risks and benefits associated with her religious involvement as these issues arise. Review with her Fallot's (2008) description of these risks and benefits. For example, therapists should be aware the role of religious delusions in psychosis and should take care not to challenge these delusions but to explore their personal meanings for women with SMI.
- Differentiate mystical, spiritual, or transcendental experiences from delusions to avoid pathologizing spiritual experiences that are culturally congruent (Mohr & Huguelet, 2006).

- Review Russinova and Cash (2007)'s descriptors of the dimensions and attitudes toward religion and spirituality among individuals with schizophrenia. This could be used as a checklist.
- Evaluate the personal meaning the woman attributes to religion and spirituality, as well as her perceived level of religiosity and spirituality. This can enhance the therapeutic alliance and help to identify the most appropriate spiritual resources to offer.
- When working with different racial-ethnic groups with SMI, be sensitive to the diversity of spiritual philosophies and religious practices across cultures, as well as the history of colonization involved in the Western influences on religion among different racial-ethnic groups.
- Encourage women with SMI to keep journals, audios, or videotapes of spiritual stories in association with their mental health journeys. In these journals, they can describe or draw metaphors of their spiritual path. Drama therapy can also be used to act out these narratives, to play music, share drawings, read, or sing with a group of people who can witness and share in these experiences (Briggs & Dixon, 2013).
- Encourage women with SMI to engage in spiritual practices that are meaningful for them. These practices could include prayer, meditation, yoga, breath work, guided imagery, tai chi, labyrinth walking, sweat lodge ceremonies, community chanting and drumming, candle lighting, or more structured prayers (Briggs & Dixon, 2013).

DISCUSSION QUESTIONS

1. Some might attribute to paranoia the reports of discrimination voiced by women with SMI. When might it be difficult to verify these perceptions, and how might clinicians handle reports of discrimination that are unclear in this way?
2. Is it appropriate to raise consciousness about racism, classism, and sexism in a psychotherapy session? Why or why not? If so, how?
3. What are your experiences with religion and spirituality, and how do you differentiate the two? How might your personal experiences shape your expectations and reactions to the spiritual and religious experiences of a woman with SMI? How could you navigate your personal biases in these areas?

ACTIVITIES

1. Spiritual Genogram. Create a spiritual genogram (Briggs & Dixon, 2013; Frame, 2000; Hodge, 2001) for yourself or someone you are working with. Use color-coding to mark the religious affiliations of family members in the diagram, note significant spiritual events within the family, and use different line thicknesses and double-headed arrows to indicate the strength of the spiritual bond between family members (Figure 6.1).

2. Spiritual Journey Narrative. Create a metaphorical story of the spiritual path in mental health (Briggs & Dixon, 2013) of yourself or someone you are working with. This could be done through a journal entry, an audio recording, a videotape, or a live performance.

3. Double Stigma and Explanatory Models. Do a little research to understand the explanatory model of mental health challenges in another country. What kinds of stigma or resilience factors are associated with that culture's mental health views? Now identify the dominant cultural attitudes toward women in that group. What does this research tell you about the potential for intersectional stigma for women with SMI in that culture? What cultural sources of resilience might they draw from to cope?

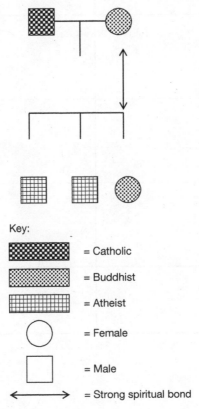

Figure 6.1 A spiritual genogram

Cultural Strengths and Stigma Worksheet

	Background/ Identification	Sources of Stigma	Sources of Resilience & Strength
Example: <u>Catholicism</u>	*Roman Catholic/ Currently non-practicing*	*Body shame, internalized homophobia*	*Prayer and singing*
Gender: _____			
Class/ Socioeconomic Status: _____			
Race & Ethnicity: _____			
Spirituality & Religion: _____			
Sexual Orientation: _____			
Other: _____			

Trauma and Sexual Objectification of Women with Serious Mental Illness

Women and girls receive cultural messages from the media that often denigrate their intelligence, fortitude, athleticism, and leadership skills. For example, consider the average billboard, magazine, TV show, and web post. Many of these modes of cultural communication depict women as scantily clad, thin, de-faced (with only parts of their body portrayed), and without wrinkles. The culture constantly sends women messages that their worth is based on their sex appeal, which is then evaluated by the public. What is the impact of living in a culture that can be so toxic to women?

Thankfully, some researchers have called attention to this sociocultural process and named it for what it is: sexual objectification. Daily experiences of being objectified have a negative effect on women's health and well-being. *Objectification theory* was proposed in 1997 as a theoretical framework to foster understanding of the unique experiences of women who live in a society that sexualizes the female body and treats it as an object (Frederickson & Roberts, 1997; Kaschak, 1992). Objectification theory provided us a way of understanding these gendered experiences. According to this research, sexual objectification occurs quite pervasively, with women regarded as sexual objects for the use of others (Bartkey, 1990).

Sexual objectification may be experienced by women in multiple ways. It can occur via everyday experiences such as continually seeing advertisements that feature half-naked, hypersexualized women, receiving a catcall while walking down the street, or being "checked out," or in more violent forms such as rape or sexual assault. Such experiences may also lead women to take on this outsider view of their own bodies (self-objectification) and begin to see themselves as objects to be evaluated based on their appearance. It is quite common in our culture for women to be scrutinized for being "fat," for their hair, or for how their clothes accentuate certain physical attributes. Women repetitively monitor their own body so as to measure up to those standards, a practice known as "body surveillance" (Frederickson & Roberts, 1997).

Interestingly, research indicates that heightened levels of self-objectification are associated with psychological challenges such as feeling shameful about one's body; thinking a lot about one's body; having anxiety about appearance; experiencing distressing emotions; and the development of eating disorders, depression, sexual dysfunction, and substance use (Carr & Szymanski, 2011; Moradi & Huang, 2008). Other psychological outcomes that are associated with sexual objectification and self-objectification include reduced "flow" (optimal experiences or heightened motivational states, such as when one feels totally mindful while playing a sport) and diminished internal awareness (turning off physiological cues such as hunger or satiety).

Researchers have taken our understanding of sexual objectification a step further in experimental studies. One study involved an impression formation task in which a sexualized or nonsexualized woman was portrayed (Loughan, Pina, Vasquez, & Puvia, 2013). Participants indicated whether they felt the different women who were presented were at any fault for being raped. Through this study, researchers were able to understand how sexually objectifying others is more associated with victim blame, as the sexualized woman in this impression formation task was more likely to be perceived as more responsible for being raped than the nonsexualized woman.

Another experimental study of sexual objectification showed that incidental exposure to sexist cues increased state self-objectification, self-surveillance, and body shame among women, but not men (Calogero & Jost, 2011). This study also showed that these effects were specific to self-objectification and not due to other factors such as a general self-focus. Furthermore, after exposure to such experiences of sexism, women planned more future behaviors related to managing their appearance than men did.

Being valued as objects and being denied a sense of humanness can lead women to act like objects lacking humanity, or a mind. Literal objectification occurs when fewer traits that distinguish them from being inanimate objects are attributed to them and when they behave more like objects (e.g., speaking less around others) when they are aware of this objectification (Heflick & Goldenberg, 2014). This may have implications for how women and girls are socialized in this culture regarding their social roles and possibilities for identity, employment, and success. They may internalize limits on their rights to use their voice, become leaders, and ultimately develop their own psychological constructs of who or what they would like to be in our society.

Some may argue that men have become as sexualized in our culture as women; however, the literature indicates that women are still more frequently objectified and hypersexualized than men (Hatton & Trautner, 2011). When women are associated with primitive constructs that are animalistic and dehumanized, men are more willing to indicate that they might sexually harass women, rape women, and hold negative attitudes toward women who were victimized (Rudman & Mescher, 2012). Interestingly, men who are more likely to automatically dehumanize women are more likely to score higher on a rape-behavioral analogue. Though one may think that sexual objectification may be harmless, there are larger implications: A culture that has a high rate of sexual objectification of women can become more dangerous for them.

Though the sexual objectification literature continues to grow, there is still a dearth of studies and theoretical frameworks that have elucidated links between serious mental illness (SMI) and sexual objectification (Carr, Greene, & Ponce, 2015). It is important to try and understand experiences of sexual objectification among women with SMI, given the unfortunate marginalization of women with SMI. Hence, it is likely that sexually objectifying experiences are high among this population, and more understanding of this process could be particularly valuable for better conceptualization, intervention, and treatment strategies (Carr et al., 2015).

This chapter will discuss the potential implications of sexual objectification for women with SMI, the associated evidence in the literature, and the high incidence of trauma and sexual trauma in this population, which have implications for psychosocial and psychological problems. This chapter will also share two case narrative composites to highlight how sexual objectification, self-objectification, and trauma appear to impact the experience of SMI among women.

PSYCHOLOGICAL TRAUMA AND POST-TRAUMATIC STRESS DISORDER

When some people experience psychological trauma occurs, life seems to go in slow motion or to stand still while something terrifying plays out in front of them. They can even dissociate, as a way for the body to care for itself in an experience that their mind has no script for. It becomes hard to grasp what has happened to them and how to explain to themselves such a shocking experience, leaving them shaken. Ultimately, such experiences, not surprisingly, leave a mark for many people. In the psychology literature, psychological trauma is defined as experiencing an uncontrollable event that is perceived or understood as an overwhelming threat to an individual's survival or sense of integrity (Herman, 1992; Mueser, Rosenberg, Goodman, & Trumbetta, 2002; van der Kolk, 1987). The American Psychiatric Association (2013) defined trauma as a stressor that an individual is exposed to, such as sexual violation, actual or threatened serious injury or death, or indirect exposure (hearing that a close friend or relative was exposed to an event; if it involved actual or threatened death, it must have been violent or accidental), witnessing a traumatic event in person, or repetitive or extreme indirect exposure to gruesome details of such traumatic events, typically in the realm of being a professional (first responders, repetitively hearing stories of child abuse). Typical forms of trauma might be violence in the form of sexual or physical assault, a traumatic death of a loved one, natural disasters, exposure to combat, or witnessing the traumatic harm of another individual (Mueser et al., 2002).

Prevalence rates of trauma exposure among the general population are consistently reported as quite high in the United States at about 90% (Breslau et al., 1998; Kilpatrick et al., 2013). Post-traumatic stress disorder (PTSD) involves experiencing a traumatic event (as just defined) that is also associated with mental health symptoms such as trying to avoid experiences associated with the trauma, re-experiencing the trauma (e.g., nightmares or flashbacks), having negative cognitions or distressing feelings, and experiencing increased arousal (feeling jumpy or on alert) (American Psychiatric Association, 2013). Prevalence rates of PTSD in the United States among the general population are about 6.8%, which is higher than that of most other countries (Kessler et al., 2008). Rates of trauma appear to be even higher among individuals who experience SMI: As many as 98% have been exposed to at least one traumatic event, with an average of 3.5 different types of traumatic lifetime exposures (Mueser et al., 1998). The prevalence of PTSD in the SMI population is also elevated in comparison to the general population, with reported rates of 29% to 43% (Mueser et al., 2002).

The literature suggests that individuals with SMI not only experience more exposure to trauma but also are at increased risk of developing PTSD in comparison to the general population (Mueser et al., 2002). To add to this concern, rates of PTSD are higher among women overall, and some of this may be due to their greater exposure to the types of trauma that are most likely to lead to PTSD, such as interpersonal assault, sexual abuse, and childhood sexual abuse (Breslau, Chilcoat, Kessler, Peterson, & Lucia, 1999). Women with SMI have also been found to have high incidence of intimate partner violence: 21% of 254 female psychiatric inpatients experienced marital rape and 42% experienced physical abuse (Cole, 1988). In another study, 26% of a sample of women who had been admitted to a psychiatric hospital had been physically abused by their male partners (Bryer et al., 1987). Thus, women with SMI may be at extreme risk of developing PTSD.

TRAUMA AND SMI

The literature indicates that trauma rates are consistently high across diverse experiences of SMI. These individuals are similarly impacted by the same type of stressors (i.e., traumatic), which are affected by the environment, from experiences with other people, and in distressing situations (Mueser et al., 2002). Trauma among individuals who experience SMI is associated with a higher incidence of substance use, more use of crisis treatment services, and greater severity of psychiatric symptoms. However, the literature is still sparse regarding how trauma specifically affects the course of illness and what treatment methods are effective. Further research is required to test whether proposed interactions of trauma and the course of SMI differ across disorders. We have found in our clinical experiences that trauma plays a major role in the development of specific symptoms and appears to be a leading factor in hospitalizations. For example, in the context of severe dissociative episodes in relation to untreated trauma, delusional states may reflect traumatic content such as the belief that one is being raped again, or feelings of paranoia that someone may hurt the person again. It is as a result of such clinical experiences that we wanted to explore the impact of trauma among this population.

WOMEN WITH SMI AND TRAUMA

Though rates of trauma are high among both men and women with SMI, there are differences across gender in the experience of different types of trauma. Women with SMI are more likely to have experienced sexual abuse (acute forms of sexual objectification) as a child in comparison to men (52% vs. 35%) (Mueser et al., 1998). Adult women with SMI report higher rates of sexual abuse than men (64% vs. 26%). Though rates of PTSD are very high, individuals with SMI have a less than 1% chance of being diagnosed with PTSD or effectively treated. As clinicians, we feel this is a social justice issue. Trauma is all too often overlooked in treatment or attributed to other symptoms such as psychosis, when, in fact, trauma is likely to impact the experience of psychosis or other symptoms. Therefore, we must accurately understand the impact of trauma so we can appropriately assess and provide sound treatment.

One may think men experience physical assault more than women, but the rates of physical assault are quite similar for men and women (Mueser et al., 2004). For example, studies among women with schizophrenia show that between 60% and 76% experienced childhood physical abuse (Friedman & Harrison, 1984; Goodman et al., 1999). What is the implication of such traumatic experiences on the occurrence of schizophrenia, and why has this been overlooked for so many years? It is quite evident to us in our clinical work that trauma plays a huge part in the content of the most defining aspects of schizophrenia, such as hallucinations and delusions.

Perhaps because women with SMI have high rates of sexual trauma, they are more likely to experience homelessness, substance use, and increased psychiatric symptoms (Goodman et al., 1995; Stein, Leslie, & Nyamathi, 2002). It has also been posited that these experiences are related to women's ability to access and engage in treatment (Goodman, Rosenberg, Mueser, & Drake, 1997). As we have observed in our clinical work, research shows that adult sexual abuse in women has been shown to be associated with hallucinations (Read, Agar, Argyle, & Aderhold, 2003). Childhood sexual abuse has been linked to delusions and thought disorders as well. Trauma in SMI is linked to more severe psychiatric symptoms with the development of PTSD (McFarlane et al., 2001).

Though there is evidence of the deleterious impact of extreme forms of sexual objectification and trauma on the lives of women with SMI, there is a gap in the scientific literature showing these connections and making recommendations for clinical practice (Carr et al., 2015). There have been some theoretical links provided in the scientific literature between sexual objectification and dissociation, suicidality, self-harm, emotion dysregulation, interpersonal effectiveness, hypervigilance, and psychosis. However, these findings need to be more thoroughly researched. It is likely that women with SMI also experience a higher incidence of everyday (insidious) sexual objectification than other women in the general population, impacting the complexity of their experience of SMI. Similarly, the intersections of multiple oppressive experiences, such as stigma related to one's mental health diagnosis, racism, poverty, sexism, and classism, may be especially challenging for these women (Carr et al., 2015; Cole, 2009; Szymanski & Moffit, 2012). To shed light on how sexual objectification and self-objectification, as well as the intersectionality of various social identities, may impact the experiences of women with SMI, a few composite narratives of the lives of women will be shared. Clinical applications will be provided to add resources for clinicians in working with women with SMI who have such experiences.

CASE NARRATIVES

Case 1: Veronica

"Veronica" is a Russian woman and immigrant in her early 30s who presented to a psychiatric inpatient unit after a suicide attempt. She had eight prior suicide attempts and a chronic history of self-injurious behavior. Typically, she would cut herself on the arms with razor blades. She had a diagnosis of borderline personality disorder in her charts, but complex PTSD appeared to be a better fit; this diagnosis captured more of her trauma history and resultant trauma symptoms, major depression with psychotic features, alcohol use disorder, and history of bulimia nervosa.

Veronica started feeling depressed in childhood and began cutting around the age of 13. This occurred a month after a 25-year-old neighbor raped her when she was playing at a friend's house. Veronica said she had told her mother at the time, but her mother did not believe the rape happened, so it was not reported to the authorities. Veronica gained a lot of weight at that point, as she engaged in overeating as a way to manage her distressing emotions. She shared that gaining the weight felt protective because men "checked her out" less, so she could guard against further assaults. However, she remembered that her self-esteem plummeted when the boys at school called her rude names about her weight gain. This started a pattern of binge eating followed by purging behavior as she tried to avoid and numb her emotions related to the rape while also attempting to live up to cultural standards of beauty.

As an adult, Veronica had two further experiences of sexual victimization. One incident occurred at a college party in which she was too drunk to consent. Another occurred when a boyfriend came back to her apartment after she had declined sexual intercourse and forced himself on her. Veronica had two or three flashbacks a week and disturbing nightmares, but her trauma had mostly gone unaddressed in her various treatment experiences.

Veronica engaged in chronic alcohol abuse as a mechanism to help her "forget" some of the horrific experiences she had endured. She had feelings of being "unlovable" and feelings of self-hate because she felt used by the world. Veronica endorsed many symptoms of depression, as well as ruminating thoughts that focused on how unattractive she was, how "fat" she felt, and how she was "ugly." Veronica engaged in daily body monitoring and surveillance as she focused on her inability to measure up to not only cultural standards of beauty, but her own internalization of those standards. Similarly, she struggled with her identity and at times of desperation had challenges with suicidal thoughts, which preceded her suicide attempts.

Veronica's case illustrates the impact of both insidious and acute forms of sexual objectification on the health and well-being of women. Similar to the literature, Veronica's experiences of acute forms of sexual objectification led to severe psychiatric impairment and suicidality. As seen in the research literature, her experiences of her depression, substance use, eating-disordered behavior, and self-objectification have been empirically correlated to experiences of sexual objectification. Therefore, Veronica's story should be understood from this sociopolitical context. Instead of taking a pathologizing individualistic stance, we must understand her current problems in the context of the environment in which she has had to survive. Furthermore, therapeutic intervention should be conceptualized from this viewpoint in order to empower the individual, deconstruct the environmental nature of the problem, increase the individual's capacity for survival, and enhance a positive sense of self.

In the clinical work with Veronica, the therapist opened up a space to assess for her trauma symptoms. Veronica was surprised that this was being addressed in her treatment as it had not been previously addressed. They discussed her treatment plan and how to help Veronica to have better coping methods to manage her suicidal ideation, parasuicidal behavior, and depression. Collaboratively, they decided to use a dialectical behavior skills therapy group approach to develop more coping strategies to regulate the distressing emotions that had led to her suicide attempts, substance use, and disordered eating. They agreed that once she increased her capacity to deal with distressing emotions in more effective ways, they would address the trauma more directly. In the meantime, they agreed to integrate cognitive strategies that were specifically helpful to her trauma symptoms and depression. These strategies included grounding techniques and engaging in behavioral activities that were soothing. Coping skills also focused on boosting positive emotions and decreasing her depressive mood state. Other exercises involved examining and reframing cognitive distortions and her cognitive schemas related to her feelings of self-worth, shame, and self-directed negative thought processes.

Next, Veronica was able to examine feelings of poor self-worth due to her traumatic experiences and feeling like she could not measure up to standards of beauty. Veronica engaged in a gender role analysis with her therapist and explored the messages she had received from the broader culture. She recognized that she believed some of her traumatic experiences were her fault. She also was concerned that she did not measure up to sociocultural standards of beauty. She was able to recognize that the content of her auditory hallucinations reflected how she had felt about herself, with voices that told her, "You're an ugly bitch" or "You might as well end it all." With support, she was able to identify that deep within herself she knew she was not to blame for her traumatic experiences. Yet the problem was with not only the individuals who had violated her, but with a society that could foster such behavior. The therapist was able to depathologize the experience of having PTSD. She reframed her difficulty processing events that were so overwhelming and gained an awareness of how her mind adapted to cope with abnormal situations.

Veronica was also able to explore the pros and cons of continuing to work so hard to examine her body to see if it conformed to society's standards of beauty. She realized how such views had impacted her experiences of depression, self-blame for traumatic experiences, auditory hallucinations, disordered eating behaviors, and substance use. While acknowledging it would be a very hard process to shift her thinking, she was able to develop her own self-defined values to determine her worth as a woman. Part of those values involved her belief that she was a beautiful person because she was intelligent, funny, and creative and cared about other people. Once she was discharged from the hospital, she was able to pursue some hobbies that she had let go in the midst of her depression, such as a creative dance group and a weekly poetry slam night. The poetry slam also gave her a place to voice some of her newly generated or revitalized beliefs and feel empowered and heard by others.

She continued to participate in the skills group in order to have positive methods for managing challenging affect, which had previously led to suicidality. Once she had a period of health and sobriety, she was able to engage in cognitive processing therapy, a cognitive intervention to address specifics related to her traumatic experiences. Engaging in therapy helped her to validate her experiences and engage in a dialogue geared at reexamining objectifying experiences as affected by her sociocultural environment. Therapy helped to shift her worldview, increase her coping, and treat the impact of the traumatic experiences she experienced. Although she had engaged in mental health services before, this was the first experience that helped her reconceptualize such traumatic experiences, leading to a redefinition of the self, a decrease in self-objectification and shame, and empowerment to engage in specific evidence-based treatment for her PTSD symptoms.

Case 2: Patrice

"Patrice" is an African American woman in her early 40s who worked as a cashier at a department store and also experienced psychosis. She reported that she lost her parents and brother in a terrible car accident at age 15. She was also in the car and had to be hospitalized for two months due to her injuries. She was so traumatized that she did not speak for three months following the incident. After this incident, she went into foster care because no one in her extended family had the resources to care for her at the time. Patrice had to live with three different families; she really enjoyed one of them, but the other two were quite distressing. In one of these homes there were two older adolescent boys who frequently made sexual comments about her body. At one point one of the boys attempted to touch her chest and genitalia, without her permission. As a result, she felt on guard and unsafe in this home.

In later adolescence and as a young woman, she realized the power of her physical body and recognized that she received a lot of attention because of her appearance. Patrice put more and more energy into maintaining her looks because she felt valued for her attractiveness, which also helped numb some of her feelings of loneliness and loss due to the family tragedy. Patrice shared that she watched what she ate, which led to frequent diets, and evaluated her appearance daily so she could continue to be the "hot girl." Patrice also talked about being aware that her attractiveness was a powerful thing in her life, but also one she associated with risk, as in several instances men had made inappropriate advances toward her, which she had to work to avoid. Such experiences made her hypervigilant and fearful of her surroundings when she went out.

In her 20s, Patrice attended college. She developed a steady boyfriend whom she loved dearly and who became the father of her child. However, after he left her, she developed more challenges. Memories resurfaced about the loss of her family, which she thought she had moved past. She began to hear voices that told her it was her fault that her family died and that her boyfriend left her. Eventually, her voices also became command hallucinations telling her to kill herself. Patrice began feeling paranoid and would lock herself in her apartment for a week at a time with her daughter in the belief that her White neighbors, who had previously made racist remarks to her on a few occasions, were trying to take her daughter. She frequently called the police and claimed that these neighbors were trying to kidnap her child. She became worried that someone was getting into their apartment and sprinkling their food with poison. Patrice started restricting what she and her daughter would eat, as well as the methods in which the food had to be sealed.

Her apartment complex manager became concerned about Patrice and the care of her daughter and called a mobile crisis unit and the police to check on them. She was then involuntarily hospitalized for an acute psychotic episode and had on-and-off custody of her daughter for the next several years. Patrice had multiple hospitalizations before she worked with a therapist and psychiatrist long term, both of who helped her gain some stability. They worked with Patrice from a trauma-informed care perspective, using ecological and interpersonal strategies that could make her feel safer while in the hospital. These elements included providing ample personal space, using language that was respectful, avoiding seclusion and restraint, and other techniques such as comfort rooms.

Patrice's individual therapist was able to address her life history and traumas. Patrice admitted she had not really gotten over this, and the loss of her family at such a young age was terrifying. As her symptoms improved with medications and she increased in her ability to reality test, she was also able to make connections between her traumatic experiences and the beliefs she had developed as part of her experience of psychosis. She felt fearful that something terrible would happen to her again and would take away the most meaningful part of her life, her daughter. The therapist created a treatment plan including developing safety strategies to manage delusions that had traumatic content. Reality testing methods were also included so she could determine whether something she thought was happening was in actuality occurring. Grounding and other personally identified strategies were used to boost her sense of empowerment and safety. A therapeutic space was also held to process her grief related to the loss of her family.

With support, Patrice began to relate that her experiences of racism also made her more paranoid around White people, thus feeling fearful that her neighbors would try to take her daughter. The therapist was able to respectfully discuss how both racism and sexual objectification had impacted Patrice during her life. Patrice noted how these oppressive experiences were very challenging and diminished her self-worth, making her hypervigilant in the broader cultural society. She felt validated by her therapist regarding these experiences and identified strategies to mitigate the impact of these oppressive experiences. Over time, she regained custody of her child and obtained a steady job again.

Similar to Veronica's story, Patrice's experiences of sexual objectification and trauma were connected to psychiatric impairment. Notably, the impact of living in a culture that treats women as sexual objects had its impact on Patrice. She began to engage in self-objectification practices such as habitual body monitoring while also having to be hypervigilant of her safety in an unsafe environment.

These case composites provide examples of how sexual objectification and trauma have a profound impact on the lives of women with SMI and the presentation of the SMI. In our clinical work with women, we have found repetitive themes of trauma, objectification, and self-objectification that appear to impact the onset of symptoms, their acuity, and the likelihood that the woman will abuse substances to self-medicate or repress disturbing traumatic emotional material. We have seen firsthand how the various social identities of these women with regard to race, poverty, and homelessness create intersecting experiences of oppression. From a feminist and recovery-oriented perspective, we must bring greater attention to the impact of sexual objectification and trauma in the lives of women with SMI. It is time to recognize the toxicity of sexual objectification in these women's lives.

CLINICAL APPLICATIONS

The high incidence of sexual objectification and traumatic experiences among women with SMI has clinical implications. First, the experiences of sexual objectification and trauma should be assessed when women initially come in for treatment. this should be done in a way that is nonthreatening and responsive to their comfort level at that stage. It is important to evaluate for any self-injurious behaviors and address those first, given the associations with sexual assault and self-harm in the literature (Rose, 1993; van der Kolk, 1994). Raising awareness of the prevalence of sexual objectification and trauma among women who have had similar mental health experiences may empower them to open up about their own experiences. A semistructured interview format for specific events or experiences may be most helpful for gathering a trauma history. Again, interviewing should be completed in the way she prefers at and a speed that is comfortable for her (Spielvogel & Floyd, 1997). It is best to obtain explicit permission from an individual to assess for trauma. It is also wise to share the limits of confidentiality and how such information will or will not be used (e.g., treatment team, family members).

Women can be engaged in gender role analyses with their clinicians to assess how they have been impacted by cultural gender messages that lead to self-objectification (Enns, 2004; Szymanski, Carr, & Moffitt, 2011; Worrell & Remer, 2003). Conversations about the impact of cultural beauty ideals on the wellness of women can be explored. Women can develop their own positive identities and engage in adaptive health-related behaviors. This discussion should be conducted with reference to the woman's other presenting symptoms, as well as her social identities and cultural background. This discussion can be strategically timed to maximize safety, coupled with the development of skills to deal with triggering discussions regarding sexually objectifying or traumatic experiences.

Women who have SMI and trauma should also be assessed for the presentation of PTSD, which is frequently overlooked (Cusack, Grubaugh, Knapp, & Frueh, 2006). If there is a presentation of PTSD, a treatment plan should be developed that targets how and when it is appropriate to treat the PTSD symptoms in relation to the woman's other diagnoses and presenting mental health symptoms. In fact, in dealing with post-traumatic stress, the timing of specific interventions may be paramount for a woman's well-being. It is a mistake to approach trauma-related material haphazardly because that may lead to the intensification of the affect and physiological states associated with the trauma and may induce other challenging behaviors that the woman may have developed as a method of adaptation (e.g., substance use, suicidality, parasuicidal behavior) (van der Kolk, 1989). Hence, it is crucial to manage other secondary behaviors and distressing affects in less harmful manners before focusing treatment directly on trauma content. Tailoring treatment to each woman's individual needs, with frequent reassessment, is crucial. Every woman has a unique story and different ways in which she has been impacted by traumatic experiences (Mueser & Taylor, 1997). A strong case formulation is essential in understanding the interaction of psychosis and post-traumatic symptoms, including risk issues, goals, and strengths (Larkin & Morrison, 2006).

There is substantial evidence to support the effectiveness of cognitive-behavioral treatments, including elements of emotional processing (Foa & Street, 2001). Dialectical behavior therapy may be helpful to increase coping with distressing affect states and other secondary behaviors such as parasuicidal behavior, which may be related to the trauma (Linehan, 1999). One of the most salient aspects of cognitive treatments is helping individuals understand that trauma reactions are normal reactions to abnormal situations rather than pathological (Reilly, 1997).

In line with recovery-oriented care, women who experience SMI and who also have PTSD should be able to engage in treatments that are evidence based for the presentation of PTSD and any SMI diagnoses (Davidson, 2009). One example of this kind of treatment is a 12-session therapeutic intervention called *Trauma Affect Regulation: Guide for Education and Therapy* (TARGET) (Ford, 2007). TARGET is listed in the Substance Abuse and Mental Health Services Administration's national registry of evidence-based practices (SAMSHA, 2012). TARGET aids individuals in the development of seven skills: focus, recognize triggers, emotion self-check, evaluate thoughts, define goals, options, and make contributions. These skills empower individuals who have experienced trauma to increase their affect regulation, to manage intrusive trauma memories, to heighten self-efficacy, and to engage in recovery.

There are many interventions to help women deal with trauma and psychiatric symptoms, such as stress management techniques (relaxation and systemic desensitization), cognitive restructuring (examining maladaptive thought patterns and establishing more adaptive thoughts), psychoeducation and behavioral family therapy (increased understanding of the experience of psychiatric symptoms and trauma, as well as development of enhanced communication skills), and social skills training (e.g., assertiveness, conflict resolution, and basic conversational skills) (Dobson & Dozois, 2010; Meuser & Taylor, 1997).

When women enter the mental health system, and especially an inpatient psychiatric unit, their trauma history and preferences should be noted in an attempt to avoid treatments that might retraumatize them (e.g., seclusion/restraints, meeting alone in a closed room with someone of the opposite gender, being around other residents who might be threatening) (Ko et al., 2008). Other options should be offered for women who have had traumatic experiences, and treatment plans should incorporate more trauma-sensitive methods. The prevention of retraumatization in trauma-informed care for women with SMI is addressed in greater detail in Chapter 8.

The oppressive experiences related to multiple social identities should be explored to understand how these layers of multiple experiences impact well-being (e.g., an African American woman with lower socioeconomic status). As multicultural feminist therapists, we believe it is important to work from a collaborative, egalitarian approach in efforts to level power differentials and since women with SMI have historically been marginalized and disenfranchised (Worell & Remer, 2000). We argue that such an approach may foster increased autonomy and a corrective emotional experience for these women, who have likely been disempowered in many mental health care and community settings. Sexually objectifying and traumatic experiences should also be considered in the context of culture, as the personal is political (Worell & Remer, 2003). Some researchers-practitioners in trauma emphasize that their work and endeavors should be examined in the light of the social, political, and economic context of the time period (Reilly, 1997). In a similar manner, trauma responses or mental health symptoms, such as the symptoms that make up PTSD diagnoses, should be conceptualized as a normal response to an aberrantly abnormal situation rather than framed as psychopathology (Reilly, 1997).

Frequently, women with SMI are treated in the public sector in outpatient and inpatient agencies that have limited resources. Though there are some evidence-based interventions to address issues of trauma and other intersecting oppressive experiences, in these settings there may be limited opportunities for staff to receive training in the clinical services that are efficacious for this population. It is important to think about how resource-limited organizations can still offer these services. Some agencies have been able to find free trainings and materials online via organizations like SAMSHA. Others have reached out to trainers of specific evidence-based treatments who can come in and train staff pro bono. Agencies have applied for grants to advance their own training and the services they can offer. Though resources may be limited in many organizations, women with SMI still have the right to receive such services. In fact, we have predominantly offered services in the public sector within organizations that have limited resources while serving the underinsured and those who experience socioeconomic disadvantages.

From a social justice and multicultural feminist perspective, we believe that intervention should not just occur at the micro-level with the individual, but should be seen as a political issue requiring political solutions (Reilly, 1997; Szymanski et al., 2011). There is a need for policies within our systems of care that relate to considerations of trauma experiences, including individuals who may have survived abuse and have to be treated for their experience of SMI in inpatient settings in which they may be further retraumatized by use of seclusions and restraints (Reilly, 1997; Wisconsin Coalition on Advocacy, 1994). Concerns related to increased allocation of resources to treat trauma among those with SMI need to be addressed at the policy level (Reilly, 1997).

Reilly (1997) also shared that exclusively political or therapeutic approaches to experiences of abuse and trauma are not sufficient and can be seen as reductionistic and unsatisfactory. The experiences of women with SMI and trauma should not be reduced to a paradigm of symptoms needing individual treatment or to the sum of one's experience with political, economic, or social forces that need large-scale political engagement to change. Instead, a broader social context needs to be engaged. This can be done by improving the mental health system, sometimes through litigation, as well as through the lens of sociopolitical contexts and historical circumstances, with a vision that acknowledges the role of power in abusive behavior that destigmatizes the impact of trauma and abuse. This holistic perspective should allow individuals to address their own situations with empowerment and support from clinicians and peers and may be able to bridge gaps between political and clinical standpoints of the problem. For example, the onus of change should be placed not on women but rather on the social norms that sexually objectify women and condone rape (Reilly, 1997; Stephan, 1995).

CONCLUSION

Women with SMI often have a history of sexual objectification and trauma. These women may have increased mental health concerns due to these experiences. The mental health system and providers need to continue to work toward meeting the diverse needs of these women and mitigating the deleterious impact of such sociopolitical experiences so women can successfully engage in their recovery.

CLINICAL STRATEGIES

The following clinical strategies are provided to help elucidate how to engage in clinical practice that is respectful of the experiences of sexual objectification and trauma in the lives of women. The strategies are meant to be used in counseling or psychotherapy encounters, given their potentially triggering nature.

- Inquire about women's sociocultural experiences of sexual objectification. Such experiences might include being evaluated by people via objectifying gaze in society to see how their "bodily goods" measure up, getting yelled at when walking down the street in relation to their body, inappropriate sexual advances, or more acute experiences such as sexual harassment, assault, or rape. Ask women how these experiences may have impacted their life and mental health.
- When women share experiences of objectification and acute forms, such as sexual harassment, assault, or rape, provide a space where they can share these in a manner that validates that such experiences are not justifiable. It can be empowering to recognize that the problem originates from society. Create space to understand how their current challenges may stem from a toxic culture, as sometimes women are given the incorrect message that they may be to blame for their experiences of victimization.
- During intake sessions, assess for a diagnosis of PTSD, as this is often overlooked and can be a result of the alarmingly high incidence of trauma among women with SMI. Use a semistructured interview format to obtain a full trauma history. Ensure that treatment of PTSD is well integrated into the treatment plan. Consider treatments that have shown efficacy for treating PTSD such as cognitive-behavioral therapy interventions that normalize aspects of trauma responses, incorporate emotional processing of memories, and address beliefs and schemas about oneself and the world.
- Inquire about experiences of sexual objectification in our culture, such as concerns about one's body size or shape, in accordance with the specific case history of each individual. Ascertain if experiences of

being objectified in our culture may impact how women may feel about themselves and their life experience. Seek ways to empower women to question the right of culture to project how a woman should define herself. Empower women in their right to take up space and feel affirmed for their worth.

- Conduct a gender role analysis (Worell & Remer, 2003) of how one's gender identity has developed and been shaped by one's culture and its impact on psychological wellness. This can involve exploring the costs and benefits of conforming to gender role expectations, as well as making decisions about behaviors that the individual may want to continue or give up. For example, some women internalize a sociocultural view of beauty standards that they need to be thin and light-skinned in order to be beautiful. Helping women question the messages they are given in society may empower them to see how society has impacted them, and how they may choose to redefine their own sense of beauty that is not distorted by an unhealthy culture.
- Encourage women to create a list of characteristics that are meaningful to them in their identity as women. Help them to understand where they developed those beliefs and to question ones that may be destructive.
- Use an example from the media, such as commercials or magazines, to help women explore the culture of sexual objectification. Support women in making healthy choices related to ingestion of messages from the media, such as finding TV shows, magazines, music, and literature that are not sexually objectifying and offer more positive messages for women.
- Explore how sexually objectifying experiences may intersect with experiences of stigma related to mental health and women's diverse social identities such as race/ethnicity, sexual orientation, age, and social class. Explore how the intersection of multiple oppressive experiences may be more intense than just one experience for a woman.
- Embolden women to engage in social justice and become involved in activism against sexual objectification of women. These activities might include encouraging women to avoid spending their money in places that sexually objectify women, writing a letter to a senator about decreasing objectification in society, or demonstrating for harsher repercussions for events such as rape on college campuses.
- Provide education about safety and crisis support to prevent sexual traumatization and to increase awareness of the appropriate resources.
- Integrate stress management techniques into psychotherapeutic experiences, such as relaxation techniques like progressive muscle relaxation, guided imagery, and visualization.
- Incorporate cognitive interventions such as cognitive restructuring by use of worksheets to combat negative automatic thoughts and provide reframes to increase healthier cognitive schemas.

- Provide social skills training, which can increase women's assertiveness, communication abilities, and boundary setting.
- Develop trainings on the impact of sexual objectification for women in your own organization, school, or system. Include information and guidelines on personal rights to ensure women are valued, respected, and empowered.
- Consider integrating family members in care through psychoeducational experiences geared at better understanding mental health. Behavioral family therapy or connections to support groups via the National Alliance on Mental Illness (NAMI) are good options.

DISCUSSION QUESTIONS

1. A common tenet of multicultural feminist therapy is the feminist motto "The personal is political." Do you agree with this conceptualization? How might this idea shape the experience of women with SMI who have encountered sexual objectification and trauma?
2. The multicultural feminist literature argues that clinicians and society must intervene at political, economic, and social levels to bridge gaps between what the individual experiences and the true historical climate in which the individual is living. What are your thoughts about this holistic approach? How do you see yourself getting involved at multiple levels? How does multilevel intervention mitigate the message individuals receive that they just have to accept and adapt to a culture that endorses sexual objectification and violence?
3. How can graduate schools, researchers, scholars, administrators, mental health systems, and clinicians work toward both the advancement of the research base and delivery of better treatment interventions to target the experience of both SMI and trauma? How do you envision being a part of this advancement?

ACTIVITIES

The following activity is meant to be an educational experience to evaluate the messages that are consumed in society. In dyads, brainstorm the following ways cultural socialization affects women with experiences of sexual objectification and trauma. Then discuss as a group the things that made the most impact on you in a culture that sexualizes the female body.

1. What messages are given to women in our culture about their body in terms of some of the following areas?
   - Body size
   - Shape

- Height
- Weight
- Skin tone
- Sexuality

2. What cultural messages justify the objectification of women? Think about how these messages are communicated in some of these arenas:
   - College campuses
   - Nightclubs
   - Sexually objectifying employment (e.g., Hooters, strip clubs)

3. What are potential ways these messages impact women and girls in the following areas? Add at least two or three other items that are not on the list.
   - Eating habits
   - Exercise
   - Skin color (including tanning, skin bleaching, colorism)
   - Dress
   - Hobbies

4. How do these messages affect women and their mental health in the following ways?
   - Mood
   - Self-esteem
   - Substance use
   - Confidence
   - Diet
   - Relationships with others

5. Where do women receive these sexually objectifying messages in society? How can we become social change agents in the following areas?
   - At school
   - In the community
   - In political arenas
   - In clinical interventions

Gender Role Analysis Worksheet

Messages About Women: What cultural messages do women receive about how they should act or look?	Cultural Differences: How do these messages differ based on age, race, ethnicity, class, or sexual orientation?
Origin: Where do these messages come from?	Oppression: How do societal standards for women harm them?
Pros: What are the advantages when women live up to these standards?	Cons: What are the disadvantages when women do not live up to these standards?
Overcoming: How can women reduce the impact of burden of cultural expectations on their lives?	Reflection: What have you learned or reinforced in completing this exercise?

8

Preventing Retraumatization
of Women with Serious
Mental Illness

Women with serious mental illness (SMI) often present to mental health settings to address psychological problems that have either developed or worsened as a result of exposure to traumatic violence and abuse. These women have a high likelihood of trauma, with some statistics estimating that as many as 51% to 97% have a physical and/or sexual assault history (Goodman et al., 1997; Goodman et al., 2001; Latalova, 2014). As we addressed in the previous chapter on sexual objectification, women with SMI appear to have a high rate of encountering sexual abuse in particular, as captured in a book devoted to this topic, *Sexual Abuse in the Lives of Women Diagnosed with Serious Mental Illness* (Harris & Landis, 1997). A report on "Violence and Trauma in the Lives of Women with Serious Mental Illness" by the British Columbia Ministry of Health Services recommended that mental health care providers be trained to "provide education assisting health care providers to assess and support violence and trauma survivors, including strategies to minimize re-traumatization in the mental health system" (Morrow, 2002, p. 34). Many signs point to the importance of working in a trauma-informed manner with women with SMI in order to prevent retraumatization.

In this chapter, we will guide our readers in the prevention of retraumatization of women with SMI. To begin, an overview of the literature will establish a basis in the conceptualization of retraumatization, which is a complex phenomenon. We will discuss the importance of assessing for a past history of trauma among these women to prevent retraumatization both inside and outside of the therapy office. We will describe the factors that contribute to retraumatization of women with SMI in mental health services. Next, we will explore relevant applications of Lenore Walker's eminent feminist theory on violence toward women—a gender-sensitive approach to this work. Several case narratives from our research interviews with women with SMI will illuminate the risk of retraumatization of women in mental health settings. In these case narratives, we will also discuss the strengths women develop to recover from trauma and mental health symptoms. Last, we will apply the findings from our research to clinical work, identifying clinical strategies to prevent retraumatization of women with SMI in mental health care.

RETRAUMATIZATION

With the growing attention to the impact of trauma on mental health, the topic of retraumatization in mental health settings has been gaining recognition. Duckwork and Follette (2013) wrote a book to this topic, *Retraumatization: Assessment, Treatment, and Prevention*. They define retraumatization as the

> traumatic stress reactions, responses, and symptoms that occur consequent to multiple exposures to traumatic events that are physical, psychological, or both in nature. These responses can occur in the context of repeated multiple exposures within one category of events (e.g., child sexual assault and adult sexual assault) or multiple exposures across different categories of events (e.g., childhood physical abuse and involvement in a serious motor vehicle collision during adulthood). These multiple exposures increase the duration, frequency, and intensity of distress reactions. (p. 2)

Their definition brings attention to the repeated traumatic incidents that have led to retraumatization across the lifespan of trauma survivors. The repetition of these events contributes to the recurrence of post-traumatic symptoms. After multiple traumas, post-traumatic symptoms may return with greater magnitude. Their definition also underscores the presence of physical symptoms of somatization among retraumatized individuals, which might mask the symptoms of post-traumatic stress disorder (PTSD) and lead to erroneous diagnoses.

A leader in this area is Ann Jennings, Ph.D., the former director of Maine's Office of Trauma Services. Jennings has presented extensively on the topic of retraumatization. In a 2009 talk, she defined retraumatization as "a situation, attitude, interaction, or environment that replicates the events or dynamics of the original trauma and triggers the overwhelming feelings and reactions associated with them." Jennings proposed that retraumatization frequently occurs in care settings when an event stirs up the original trauma. This trigger might resemble the original trauma in terms of content or interpersonal dynamics. The retraumatization reaction might be obvious or might be overlooked by clinicians, partly since the survivor is often unaware of the link between the original trauma and the triggering event.

Retraumatization can also occur within an inpatient unit or other residential treatment facility; this is referred to as "sanctuary trauma." People with SMI are vulnerable to force in these settings all too often. Sanctuary trauma was a term coined by physician Steven Silver based on his work with veterans. He defined sanctuary trauma as an experience that "occurs when an individual who suffered a severe stressor next encounters what was expected to be a supportive and protective environment" (Silver, 1986, p. 215). This term has been applied to psychiatric settings in which trauma was experienced firsthand or vicariously (Frueh et al., 2000).

As we have discussed in previous chapters, individuals with SMI have an elevated prevalence of trauma in general. According to a study by Mueser and colleagues (1998), 98% of individuals with SMI reported exposure to at least one traumatic event, and 43% met criteria for PTSD as result of trauma. This study also reported high frequencies of sanctuary trauma among participants with SMI, with 8% reporting a history of sexual assault in a treatment facility, 31% reporting physical assault, and 63% having witnessed a trauma. These devastating rates speak to the grave risk of traumatization and retraumatization among people with SMI in psychiatric hospitals.

Robins and colleagues (2005) referenced William Anthony's (1993) important comments on sanctuary trauma. Anthony has been a leader of the psychiatric rehabilitation and recovery movement. He envisioned the recovery process as follows: "Recovery from mental illness involves much more than recovery from the illness itself. People with mental illness may have to recover from the stigma they have incorporated into their very being; [and] from the iatrogenic effects of treatment settings" (Anthony, 1993, p. 7). Anthony portrayed healing from the effects of sanctuary trauma as a key element of the recovery process. In his work, he addressed the excessive use of force and restraints in mental health settings that has traumatized and retraumatized individuals with SMI. Consequently, steps have been taken to put in place alternative approaches that reduce the use of restraints and other types of force given their traumatizing nature in many treatment facilities. This includes practices like the "No Force First" policy (Ashcraft, Bloss, & Anthony, 2012) that has been instituted in many inpatient settings. Unfortunately, research suggests that the use of physical force in inpatient settings and sanctuary trauma continues to be a problem that contributes to retraumatization in mental health care and requires clinical attention (Cusack, Cusack, McAndrew, McKeown, & Duxbury, 2018).

WOMEN AND RETRAUMATIZATION

Women and those with SMI are particularly vulnerable to sanctuary trauma and retraumatization given their high rates of physical and sexual violence and abuse (Chandy, Blum, & Resnick, 1996; Goodman et al., 2009). A meta-analysis of 30 years of research (Mauritz, Goossens, Draijer, & van Achterberg, 2013) confirmed that women with SMI have higher rates of sexual abuse than men (20% to 34% for men vs. 44% to 64% for women). This gender disparity is found in the general population as well, though at lower rates (14% for men, 32% for women). Furthermore, women who have encountered trauma have an increased risk of developing a mental health problem (Herman, 1997). According to one study, 46% of chronically hospitalized women with psychosis had a history of childhood incest (Beck & van der Kolk, 1987). Another study found that 55% of the women who received outpatient mental health services reported a history of childhood sexual abuse, as compared to 18% of the men (Lipschitz et al., 1996). A third study found that 53% of women who had been in an inpatient psychiatric inpatient unit reported a history of physical or sexual abuse compared to 23% of the men (Carmen, Rieker, & Mills, 1987). These findings suggest that the variables of gender, SMI, and trauma are connected in an interlocking pattern of risk.

TRAUMA ASSESSMENT

Effective detection and assessment of trauma among women with SMI is the first step to ensuring trauma-informed care for this population. When beginning a trauma assessment, it is important for clinicians to remember that people may be hesitant to disclose a trauma history, especially at the onset of treatment. It is also possible that the provider may not have assessed for trauma at all (Jennings, 2009). In some cases, reports of past and current abuse are ignored, disbelieved, discredited, or judged to be irrelevant to treatment altogether. Whether deliberate or accidental, a woman may feel her trauma is being dismissed, and she may be less likely to access care in the future.

Assessment issues in trauma-informed care for women with SMI may also involve diagnostic mislabeling by providers. In her classic work *Trauma and Recovery* (1997), the feminist psychiatrist Judith Herman discussed the implicit bias of victim blaming in the mental health field. There has been a historical tendency for providers to find problems in the character of the survivor that predisposed her to abuse or violence. Herman acknowledged that there is a legitimate possibility for psychopathology to exist prior to abuse and also to result from the abuse. Nonetheless, there is a continued tendency to focus on a woman's predisposition to abuse and violence in discussions of women's trauma. Trauma survivors may present with symptoms of anxiety, depression, somatization, psychosis, and characterological issues. However, Herman argued that this symptomatology tends to present differently among survivors of trauma.

Herman (1997) cautioned that accurate detection and diagnosis of trauma in survivors may be obscured by presenting problems that are not clearly related to trauma, such as relationship issues and self-esteem. As a result, both parties may lack awareness of the connection of these problems to trauma. Moreover, trauma survivors often have multiple diagnoses before PTSD is recognized. These symptoms might include somatization, represented by the trauma survivor's disruption of sense of body and storing of pain. The woman may be diagnosed with borderline personality disorder, due to the lack of a sense of safety in relationships and attachments without boundaries. The woman may also be diagnosed with a dissociative identity disorder due to symptoms of dissociation, disturbance in identity, and disruption of affect as a result of the trauma.

· To capture the clustering of these symptoms for survivors of repeated trauma, Hermann (1997) presented the diagnosis of complex PTSD (C-PTSD). Symptoms in the criteria list for C-PTSD include prolonged exposure to trauma, problems with affect regulation, alterations in consciousness, alterations in self-concept, and interpersonal problems. Field trials were conducted to identity clinical support for the inclusion of C-PTSD in the most recent edition of the American Psychiatric Association's *Diagnostic and Statistical Manual of Mental Disorders*, the DSM-5. However, researchers were unable to identify empirical support for the diagnosis of C-PTSD. As an alternative, some revisions were made to the criteria of PTSD to be more inclusive of Herman's proposed symptoms of C-PTSD. More research is needed to evaluate the potential diagnosis of C-PTSD (Resick et al., 2013). However, it is a valuable means of conceptualizing the complex effects of multiple traumas on the personality and symptoms of women with SMI, as well as their potential vigilance for retraumatizing experiences.

RETRAUMATIZATION IN MENTAL HEALTH SERVICES

Trauma survivors might experience revictimization by caregivers, given a tendency to engage in interactions that replicate the behavior of the perpetrator (Herman, 1997). This vulnerability includes sexual abuse by providers or by abusive peers in a treatment program, or reenactment of physical or sexual abuse-like scenarios on an inpatient unit. These scenarios may involve force-feeding, restraints, and other uses of force in psychiatric hospitals.

Jennings (2009) described the experience of retraumatization in mental health settings. As a result of the replication of trauma in mental health services, trauma survivors experience feelings of being unseen and unheard by their providers. The treatment may remind them of how they were stifled in speaking out about their abuse. They may feel blamed and shamed for their trauma by providers, as they did with their perpetrators, for not cooperating and being a "good patient" or "good victim." They may feel controlled by or powerless to confront their providers. They can feel trapped in hospitals or in provider relationships where they feel unprotected and susceptible to further abuse. They may experience violations of their right to privacy or boundaries, and may feel objectified and betrayed by their providers as they did by their perpetrators. As a result, the services that were intended to be helpful actually come to mirror their relationships with their perpetrators.

For women with SMI, further retraumatization could lead to a magnification of the cognitive symptoms of mental illness, including confusion and lack of clarity. Women with SMI may become increasingly paranoid, anxious, or fearful as a result of the triggering of the past trauma. They may also become depressed as a result of the impact on mood and sense of self, leading to hopelessness or despair. Careful attention must be paid to trauma content in delusions as there may be communication of a history of abuse in distorted thoughts about the present. Attributing the abuse solely to psychosis might feel invalidating, dismissive, and retraumatizing.

Jennings (2009) explained that people with trauma histories who have been retraumatized in mental health settings may present with diminished trust in providers and experience difficulty engaging in treatment. Retraumatization in mental health services can increase self-injurious behaviors and aggravaté the intrusive symptoms of trauma, including nightmares, flashbacks, and other re-experiencing symptoms. When these symptoms are extreme, they may take on a delusional quality. The intensity and chronicity of their symptoms can increase, both before and after discharge from inpatient or outpatient care. As a result, these women may be more likely to encounter a relapse in symptoms and re-quire rehospitalization. A revolving-door scenario can then develop where their symptoms are worsened by retraumatization in mental health settings, and then they are returned to those settings where their symptoms were triggered, risking further retraumatization.

RETRAUMATIZATION AND BARRIERS TO HELP SEEKING

Feminist therapy leader Lenore Walker has written extensively on providing mental health services for traumatized women. In her book *Abused Women and Survivor Therapy: A Practical Guide for the Psychotherapist* (1994), Walker identified the ways that abuse blocks the access to help in the first place. Retraumatization may occur because trauma poses barriers to help seeking, preventing intervention to end the abuse and putting women at risk of additional trauma. In this section, we will elucidate and apply Walker's theory to the retraumatization of women with SMI.

Abuse can lead to a sense of denial given, that the perpetrator often silences or threatens the woman, denies the occurrence of the abuse, or names the ex-perience as something other than abuse. Enablers of the abuse may have also silenced the woman or dismissed what has happened. On the other hand, de-nial may prevent distress and allow the avoidance of conflicting feelings about the abuse (Walker, 1994). The denial may also be self-protective in helping the survivor to avoid opening up the distress of the trauma. Denial can delay the treatment process until safety has been established or the client feels a sense of readiness to begin treatment. Denial may also represent a strategy to avoid di-rect confrontation with and additional aggression by the perpetrator. Finally, denial of the abuse may be culturally rooted: Denial may be used to avoid the potential shame the abuse would bring to one's family or community and to save face.

The survivor may take on a sense of responsibility for the trauma, and/or shame and guilt that interferes with accessing help (Walker, 1994). Self-blame may occur, given ideas that the perpetrator or others may have told the survivor about de-serving the abuse. The perpetrator may have deflected responsibility to the sur-vivor to maintain power. Survivors also tend to blame themselves in order to feel a sense of control over what happened to them. Western culture tends to blame victims, and self-blame may reflect an internalization of these cultural messages. Victim blaming can lead the public to remain passive instead of taking action, adding to the illusion that others are immune to violence or abuse.

Violence and abuse can produce cognitive confusion and dissociative effects that interfere with memory or clarity about what happened (Walker, 1994). This process could lead to difficulties recognizing, talking about, and naming the traumatic event. It can also lead to impaired concentration, dissociation, flashbacks, nightmares, and hypervigilance. Survivors may fear function loss from symptoms like these when addressing the trauma. Therefore, clinicians can reassure their clients that sustaining functioning would be a goal of treatment.

Another issue in trauma that can interfere with accessing help is that the survivor may fear punishment by the perpetrator (Walker, 1994). This retaliation may come directly from the perpetrating caretaker, partner, enabler, or other involved party. Retaliation may involve verbal punishment, scapegoating, or isolation. Alternatively, survivors may fear isolation from their family or community as a result of exposing the abuse to a provider.

Trauma survivors may develop "pleasing behavior" as a coping mechanism learned from the abuse in order to appease the perpetrator (Walker, 1994). Pleasing behavior may interfere with the survivor's revealing of abuse and trauma; instead, the client may focus on being a "good client" or easy for the provider to deal with. People-pleasing may have been part of the conditioning of the perpetrator's forced cooperation of the survivor with the abuse. The survivor may also have developed a people-pleasing style to satisfy the enablers of the perpetrator, such as other family members or caregivers who permitted the abuse to occur or denied its occurrence.

Finally, the client may avoid mental health treatment for trauma because of fear of provider revictimization (Walker, 1994). As we have discussed, survivors are vulnerable to sexual abuse by providers. They may fear that the provider will dismiss or deny their abuse. Walker cited the tendency of those in the mental health field to identify survivors' stories as "screen memory," delusions, and secret fantasies or wishes attributed to oedipal complexes. These ideas, which have not been supported by research, continue to blame the victim and pose barriers to help seeking.

Though Walker's work on trauma was written many years ago, her work still holds up today in understanding how trauma is reenacted in the lives of survivors of abuse. Nevertheless, there have been innovations in trauma-informed practice and theory since then, and they were the subject of a recent review (Condino, Tanzilli, Speranza, & Lingiardi, 2016). For one, we have gained a greater understanding of the traumatic nature of witnessing or learning about trauma rather than experiencing it solely firsthand. This is reflected in the modification to the definition of "traumatic incident" in the DSM-5 (APA, 2013). Initiatives have also been developed to prevent the perpetration of abuse by training children and adolescents to promote gender equality (Condino et al., 2016). Greater efforts are being made to screen people for abuse, particularly women and children, such as in the context of a visit to a primary care provider. More work is being done to target perpetrators of abuse and to end the cycle through mandatory arrest and group treatment programs, including blending of psychoeducation (i.e., the Duluth Model) with feminist and cognitive-behavioral therapy. Interpersonal, psychodynamic, and feminist therapies also continue to be used with female survivors of abuse, with greater attention to issues of intersectionality, such as including racial-ethnic, sexual, and socioeconomic factors in treatment.

As demonstrated in this section, the effects of trauma can lead to a cycle of abuse and retraumatization. In the next section, we will present several case narratives from our research interviews with women with SMI to demonstrate the nature of retraumatization among women with SMI, as well as strategies for prevention. These stories will illustrate experiences of trauma and retraumatization in the lives of women with SMI and identify ways that women draw from their strengths to access help and foster resilience.

CASE NARRATIVES

Case 1: Anna

"Anna" is a White American, Catholic lesbian woman in her 50s. She was sexually abused throughout her childhood by her mother's boyfriend. This incident was only the first of many, as she had been mistreated sexually by more people than she could recall. She was first diagnosed with PTSD at age 20 and later was diagnosed with bipolar disorder. During her younger years she was repeatedly hospitalized in psychiatric units, where she had a range of positive and negative experiences. At best, the hospital served as a refuge and offered a sense of safety from a world that felt terrifying. At worst, a hospital stay could be retraumatizing during a most vulnerable time.

Anna described a particularly challenging incident in her mental health care that occurred around the time she was being stalked by her employer. She was so triggered around her earlier sexual trauma that she developed psychotic symptoms and needed to be hospitalized:

> I had a psychiatrist tell me that I'd never have a job, I'd never have a spouse, I wouldn't work, and I was too sick for treatment, and I would only be referred out to respite care. And I love living every day proving him wrong...Doomsday predictions. You know, it was horrible what happened. Then he kicked me out of the hospital, and I was actually hiding in that hospital because I had a boss who was stalking me. And I just kept going into hospitals because it was hard for him to get to me ... So, when he discharged me without any medication and discontinued my treatment because the hospital that he worked at, he also worked at the place I was getting therapy. I started having these panic attacks and they were, like, 24/7. It was for a month or so and I thought, I was a young adult and I thought I was going crazy and I didn't know what anxiety was. I just felt like I needed people to take care of me 24/7.

It is not uncommon for people in recovery from mental illness to describe receiving pessimistic predictions from a provider who presents mental illness as a death sentence. People with mental illness have often described providers who made grim prognoses that robbed them of hope. In this case, the psychiatrist may have even lacked hope for treatment. With the added financial pressures posed by insurance companies, many of these clients are prematurely discharged.

During her hospitalization, Anna was not treated in a manner that was responsive to her history of trauma, causing retraumatization. Given her history of sexual trauma by her mother's boyfriend and her mother's failure to end it, Anna was desperate for stabilizing relationships and environments that would protect her from abuse. This retraumatization had devastating effects:

> I said, if this is going to be my life, I want to be dead. And I did this: I tried to kill myself, you know. And when it didn't happen, I kept cutting and cutting and the blood would go like this [*gesturing*], and then it would stop and I was like, why is it stopping? I finally went to the hospital and I said to my doctor, I said, "Why? How come I couldn't die? How come I couldn't bleed to death? You know, the blood was shooting out and it wouldn't stop." She goes, "Don't you know the men that go to war, they get limbs blown off and they don't die?" And I'm like, "No, I didn't know that." (*Laughs*)

Anna's experience in the hospital unwittingly reenacted her earlier abuse, leading her to suicidal behavior. Anna felt unable to live in a world that was so harmful and unsafe. She came to resemble a wounded soldier living in a war zone. In a system that felt unresponsive to her pain, she used self-harm to make her emotional pain physical.

Anna returned to the hospital and found a more healing experience. She found a psychiatrist who validated her sense of mistreatment by her previous provider. He prescribed anxiety medication that brought her relief and gave her a sense of control over the panic. Anna reflected on the traumatic nature of her first episode of psychosis and her vulnerability during her hospitalization at this time:

> The first time I went to a hospital it was very traumatic, you know. After looking back, I felt like I was so traumatized. I was put in _____ Hospital back when it was like a Club Med. I mean, it was, like, a really nice place. But still, you know, looking back, I thought a lot of psychologists there, the psychiatrists, they want to move right to the fact that you're ill. And it's almost like a first-episode psychosis. You really need to treat that feeling of shock, you know? Because it was a trauma. It was the shock and that never got tended to. And as I said, even with first-episode psychosis or early onset psychosis, we know now it's important to treat that. Anybody else that's newly diagnosed also needs that.

Later, Anna began a relationship with a woman who had been her mental health provider in a battered women's shelter. She was receiving a number of mental health services in a nearby town that she found incredibly helpful. When insurance companies threatened to cut her treatment short or redirect her to a provider closer to her in a town where her perpetrating therapist lived, Anna called in suicide threats to her insurance companies and successfully masqueraded as her psychiatrist to the insurance company to grant her more sessions. She made desperate attempts to secure the relationships and care that helped her to recover and was labeled with borderline personality disorder. She believed this diagnosis was also used by providers to understand her attraction to women:

> Again, a lot of psychiatrists [say], "That's part of the borderline personality disorder—she's confused about her sexuality." Instead of saying, "She's gay— it's a healthy part of her," they would pathologize it. I think they did pathologize it. I think it's part of [being] diagnosed with borderline personality disorder. And you know, when I went to the trauma clinic my therapist said, "You're not borderline. You have PTSD. That's not the way I would describe you." And, what happened when I went in the first hospital, I was trying to get away from that therapist. We were living together, and I wanted to get away from that therapist, so I went into the hospital and they did all these tests. And I said, "What's wrong with me?" And they said, "What's wrong with you is you're a borderline personality disordered person." And then the staff in the hospital stopped talking to me. You know, everything was at an arm's length. I knew I wasn't liked because of that label. And it really hurt my self-esteem. And instead of saying, "What's wrong with you is you're living with your therapist and that's not healthy" . . . they let that person come and visit, you know? And even touch me in, in the—you know. It was awful.

Anna was able to develop goals and supportive relationships, despite the traumatizing relationships she had in her family, with her providers. She even pursued a career as a peer specialist to support others with mental health problems:

> I've had goals and I've been able to provide myself with help, hope. And I've been able to get people to rally my cause. I have a huge support system. And, you know, I have a talent for spreading that support system out so I don't burn anyone out . . . [and] helping people build a support network. It's something that I came with. It was a talent I had but not everybody has that. You need at least five good supporters in your life when you have a mental illness.

Anna revealed a serious history of trauma alongside a number of strengths and proactive coping strategies she developed to deal with her trauma. Lacking support and trauma-responsive providers in the hospital caused her to experience abandonment by the caregivers from whom she sought help and protection. Anna also spoke to the nature of her first hospitalization and psychotic episode as traumatic in nature. As we stated earlier, research has confirmed the traumatic nature of the first episode of psychosis (Mueser & Rosenberg, 2003). Finding a provider who approached her with sensitivity to her history of trauma was essential to her recovery and helped her to become a resource in the recovery process of others.

In this next case narrative, we will see other strengths and strategies women with SMI draw from to prevent retraumatization in mental health settings.

Case 2: Raya

We return to the story of "Raya" from Chapter 6, who provides a rich portrait of issues of trauma and culture. As we previously discussed, Raya is a biracial Black and Asian bisexual, pagan woman in her 40s with a physical disability and a history of chronic pain and PTSD. Raya described herself as a survivor of childhood incest and sexual exploitation. She developed a heroin addiction at age 12 after her mother died. That was around the time she was first diagnosed with a mental health problem:

> I was diagnosed with just depression and anxiety. They weren't sure if there was such a thing as non-combat PTSD yet because it was the early [19]80s. They didn't know that people who had traumatic real-life experiences could also have PTSD.

. After her mother died, Raya began to use heroin with her stepfather as a way to cope. She and her brothers went to live in the home of a relative, and she was sexually assaulted by a family member. She turned to sex work as a source of income for herself and her brothers and to support her heroin habit. Her father was unable to care for her during those years due to his own mental health problems. Once she turned 19, she became paid by the state to be his caretaker, which continued until he died when Raya was 30. She recounted caring for her father as often traumatizing: "He was an emotionally abusive rage-a-holic, alcoholic. I had to survive him tearing me emotionally to pieces every day."

After Raya's father died, she became homeless for several years until she could obtain subsidized housing. As a result of her anxiety, physical disabilities, and chronic pain, she has been unable to pursue formal work options and subsisted on public assistance.

Raya described her impairing experiences of anxiety and pain as being transactional in nature: "My anxiety makes my pain levels worse, and it can get really bad because the more pain I get, the more anxiety I get." When she feels well enough, she fills her days with activism and psychosocial rehabilitation programs where she connects to her community of peers.

Raya finds therapy to be a vital source of support. Given her complex history of abuse, she has been savvy about identifying therapists who feel safe and appear trauma-informed:

> I choose my therapists really carefully . . . If I was going to work with someone who was male, he would have to be queer. And if I was going to work with someone who was female, I'd hope that she'd respect the background of a trauma survivor . . . It's really important to me and . . . it's part of my lead-in

questions to any therapist I have . . . I wouldn't go anywhere that didn't re-spect the fact that I was a trauma survivor. I wouldn't go to anyone who wasn't female or hadn't also worked with people with PTSD . . . with other trauma survivors, and that they have a history of actually helping ongoing trauma survivors. I look for certain books on people's bookshelves. If they don't have a couple really good survivor manuals, I won't talk to them.

Clearly, finding a trauma-informed provider is at the top of her mind when seeking a new therapist. She also selects therapists based on a number of charac-teristics that help her to feel safe as a survivor.

Raya also viewed her experience of PTSD as contributing to her resilience:

I think my strength has been the fact that I've been willing to learn more about how to control my PTSD and how not to get easily triggered. I haven't had to work since I had a full diagnosis of PTSD. But I think on a daily basis, I try not to get triggered and try to make sure I take care of myself. And I try to make sure that I'm not stressed out even though I do have a tendency to panic.

Raya's story demonstrates ways in which women with trauma histories may be vigilant about avoiding retraumatization in therapy. They may "read" their therapists for verbal and nonverbal cues of safety and competence, such as scan-ning the therapist's shelves for trauma manuals. Trauma survivors may also select therapists with characteristics they identify as safe, such as Raya's selection of gay male therapists or female therapists given her history of abuse by straight men.

Her ability to manage her symptoms of PTSD became a source of self-efficacy and resilience. Through careful selection of her therapists, she created relationships that provided a foundation of healing from the effects of family abandonment, ne-glect, and abuse. While Raya continues to struggle with anxiety and somatic pain, she has been able to maximize her coping with PTSD to enhance her quality of life and sense of self.

APPLICATIONS TO CLINICAL WORK

A number of applications to clinical work emerge from this literature to avoid the retraumatization of women with SMI in mental health care. As evidenced by these case narratives, it is essential to take a careful history of trauma and the dy-namics that reproduce these experiences. Providers can work collaboratively with survivors to establish discharge plans that are appropriate and empowering and reduce feelings of abandonment. Clinicians should make diagnoses carefully, and imbue these discussions with a sense of hope. Providers can be mindful of how first-episode psychosis may be triggered by multiple stressors in trauma survivors, and treat psychotic breaks as potentially traumatizing in nature. Clinicians can also be sensitive to ways that borderline personality disorder may stigmatize the coping strategies of survivors and brand them as "difficult." Clinicians can help these clients to build up their support networks in healing from traumatizing relationships in their past. It is important to be sensitive to ways that trauma manifests in the body, particularly around somatic pain. Clinicians can reinforce trauma survivors' careful screening of providers and investigate ways to help them feel safe and avoid reproducing traumatizing dynamics in therapy. Providers can also ensure that they achieve competence in trauma-informed work and convey this to survivors.

Other authors have made recommendations for trauma-informed care. Herman (1997) outlined ways that the relationship between the client and the provider can constitute a healing relationship that validates her experience. For one, clinicians should avoid any actions that could appear to be controlling of the client. Instead, they can help her feel empowered in managing her behavior. While clients may need to be hospitalized if their behavior is a significant risk, they should be given as much choice as possible. Clinicians should also be aware of the transference that can occur if the client places the clinician on a pedestal as the idealized "rescuer" from her trauma. Conversely, the client may transfer onto the therapist the perpetrator identity, as individuals in caregiver roles may have historically exploited them.

Walker (1994) made a number of recommendations for survivor therapy that can be applied to avoid retraumatization of women with SMI. First, the provider can provide the client with a sense of safety and feeling of being understood, given the likely history that the abuse was denied or the woman's reports were dismissed. Restoring clarity in judgment is an important part of this process, given that the perpetrator or enablers have likely challenged or neglected the survivor's feelings about the abuse. Alternatively, the symptoms of the trauma may involve distortions in thinking or confusion that could benefit from added clarity in mental health treatment. Clients may need to be gently challenged around internalized self-blame and the tendency to deem themselves responsible for the abuse.

In addition, clinicians can educate their clients on the effects of the trauma and provide treatment that effectively reduces the symptoms of the trauma (Walker, 1994). This treatment may take the form of a range of trauma-specific or more general interventions that have demonstrated benefit to trauma survivors. Interventions are being developed to tailor treatments for people with SMI and PTSD, with some positive findings for cognitive restructuring, breath training, and psychoeducation approaches (Mueser et al., 2015; Nishith, Mueser, & Morse, 2015; Steel et al., 2017). Providers can allow clients to pace themselves throughout their treatment and set their own timetable for addressing the trauma to give them a sense of control. This approach honors their self-protective instincts and defers to their readiness for addressing the trauma. Survivors may benefit from understanding the systemic nature of oppression toward women, as well as women with a SMI, given their double risk of violence. The clinician can focus on re-empowering female survivors using a strengths-based approach that instills confidence in their ability to make decisions about their lives and avoid further abuse.

Clinicians may experience a tendency to pressure survivors into forgiving their perpetrators or those who enabled the abuse. There is sometimes a view in the field that this forgiveness process is needed in order for healing from trauma to occur. Pressuring the client to forgive, however, may contribute to retraumatization. Such pressure can dismiss the client's legitimate anger toward the perpetrator. Rushing forgiveness can challenge the client's valuable survival reaction to avoid, condemn, and/or protect herself from the perpetrator.

Malcolm, DeCourville, and Belicki (2008) addressed this issue in their edited book *Women's Reflections on the Complexities of Forgiveness*. The authors explained that forgiveness research often presents this construct as positive, while the sexual abuse literature has been more ambivalent. One challenge is that there are variations in how forgiveness is defined in the literature. Ultimately, it is recommended that survivors be given the self-determination to decide if forgiveness is a goal or a desired outcome of their trauma work. The survivor should be allowed to decide when, if, or whom she forgives.

Furthermore, research suggests that forgiveness may not always be needed to ensure a positive outcome (Malcolm et al., 2008). A focus on self-repair and internal healing is more of a priority of treatment. Pushing forgiveness may interfere with achieving a healthy type of forgiveness. Maladaptive forms of forgiveness may backfire and contribute to further self-blame, passive resignation, and a return to abusive relationships.

Self-care and awareness on the part of clinicians are central to preventing retraumatization of women with SMI. Trauma therapists might experience "countertransference trauma" or vicarious trauma; as a result of listening to stories of trauma, clinicians may experience a loss of faith in therapy or humanity and nightmares, distress, contagious dissociation, dysphoric mood, or other negative effects (Herman, 1997; McCann & Pearlman, 1990). They may feel an excessive sense of responsibility, guilt, or incompetence in conducting trauma work (Herman, 1997). Providers may encounter countertransference in feeling identified with the abused client, intimidated by her, or incompetent at treating her. Providers may also experience compassion fatigue (Figley, 1995). Compassion fatigue can include apathy, isolation, and substance abuse to cope with caregiving without self-care.

Conversely, providers could experience "witness guilt," similar to survivor guilt, for not having gone through the abuse that their clients describe (Herman, 1997). Herman cautioned that countertransference may involve such bewildering experiences as identification with the perpetrator or sexual arousal that can be difficult to discuss in supervision or consultation. Problems with therapists' management of countertransference and self-care can lead to burnout and further letdown of the client.

Jennings (2009) indicated that client retraumatization has a major impact on staff and providers. Retraumatization of clients may lead to staff assault and injury, nonadherence to treatment, and consumer complaints. Staff may face stress and secondary trauma as a result of witnessing trauma on inpatient units, producing low morale and staff turnover. These factors can extend to outpatient clinicians, who may risk burnout and absenteeism. Under these conditions, clinicians might also become disengaged in treatment, less effective, and prone to producing retraumatization.

It is essential to maintain effective boundaries with clients with trauma histories (Herman, 1997). While at times the trauma may lead survivors to request leniency in boundaries, giving in and granting too much flexibility could actually feel unsafe. At other times, clinicians may feel victimized by clients, who may reenact the abusive behavior of their perpetrator or place inordinate expectations on the therapist to rescue them from the abuse. It is important to conduct formal or informal contracting with the client at the outset of services to delineate boundaries of the work and to affirm a commitment to establish safety for both client and provider. Consultation, peer supervision, and other supports are essential to conducting trauma care. As Herman stated, "no one can face trauma alone." Providers may also find it helpful to use the clinical worksheet at the end of this chapter, the "Preventing Trauma and Retraumatization Worksheet," with women with SMI or others who may benefit.

CONCLUSION

Women with SMI are at risk of retraumatization because they are both people with mental illness and women. They are particularly vulnerable to sanctuary trauma as well and may have histories of multiple traumas in mental health settings that can block access to care. Providers can ensure their competence in trauma-informed treatment and be aware of the factors that mask symptoms of trauma or interfere with help seeking. A recovery-oriented and gender-sensitive approach to clinical work with women with SMI can enhance the effectiveness of treatment and reduce retraumatization in mental health care.

CLINICAL STRATEGIES

- Seek training in trauma-informed work and communicate this competence to survivors.
- Inquire as to past histories of trauma and abuse to ensure prevention of retraumatizing dynamics in therapy.
- Ask about retraumatizing experiences in hospitalizations or with other providers.
- Explore how the survivor may experience the reenactment of traumatizing experiences in her current personal and professional relationships and in settings such as work, home, community, social network, or the treatment milieu.
- Explore with the person how the therapeutic relationship can avoid reproducing triggering or retraumatizing dynamics through transference.

- Validate the person's feelings about the trauma and gently challenge the tendency to blame herself and internalize the abuse, which can contribute to engagement in retraumatizing relationships. Help her to build insight and awareness of these tendencies.
- Provide psychoeducation on the effects of trauma and contribution to risk of retraumatization in order to increase awareness and a sense of control.
- Check in about the pacing of trauma-focused clinical work in order to prevent retraumatization and to keep the survivor from becoming "flooded" and overwhelmed.
- Avoid forgiveness pressure. Encourage survivors to take their time to decide if, when, and/or how to forgive perpetrators—if at all.
- Monitor yourself for symptoms of vicarious traumatization, hopelessness, witness guilt, fatigue, increased illness, disengagement, fear, and other potential effects of trauma work.
- Find places to gain support for countertransference reactions that can arise within you as a provider, given the potential for retraumatization in therapy. Since the provider's intention to help, the slow progress of trauma work can contribute to therapist burnout and compassion fatigue. Clinicians need to be vigilant about self-care in order to sustain this difficult but monumentally important work.

DISCUSSION QUESTIONS

1. How do multiple experiences of stigma add risk to retraumatization for women with SMI? Consider the case of women with SMI who also encounter mental illness stigma, sexism, racism, and homophobia.
2. Do you think men and women might differ with regard to their experience of retraumatization in general and in mental health settings? Why or why not? If so, in what ways?
3. What steps can be taken to reduce the risk of therapist burnout and compassion fatigue in working with trauma survivors?
4. What types of policy or social change are needed to reduce the incidence of trauma and retraumatization of women? What steps would be needed to implement that policy change?
5. Family violence has been portrayed as a public health issue and a disease that travels across communities. From this perspective, what are the causes and ripple effects of trauma on families, communities, and societies? What contributes to problems with violence in a culture and society, and what conditions and supports effectively put a stop to this violence?

ACTIVITIES

1. Research Project. Conduct a Google search on budget cuts and other problems of the deinstitutionalization movement in the treatment of people with SMI. Identify three factors in deinstitutionalization that may have contributed to the retraumatization of people with SMI in mental health settings.

2. Brochure. Create a brochure for mental health services for women with SMI. Explain in person-centered language how these services are trauma-informed, heal the effects of trauma, and prevent the risk of retraumatization.

3. Role Play. Role play a provider working with a woman with SMI who experienced retraumatization during a recent hospitalization. As the clinician, follow the clinical strategies list to conduct the session in a manner that avoids retraumatization and provides psychoeducation and validation to the survivor. Consider having a third person serve as a supervisor to the clinician who is feeling burned out in working with the client.

4. Take the Professional Quality of Life Scale (PROQOL; www.ProQOL. org) to assess your levels of Compassion Satisfaction, Burnout, and Secondary Traumatic Stress.

Preventing Retraumatization Worksheet

Mental health challenges:

Mental health strengths:

Difficult experiences that created a lack of safety:

Positive experiences that created a sense of safety:

Triggers:

Coping strategies:

Factors that make mental health services feel less safe:

Factors that contribute to a sense of safety in mental health services:

Supportive relationships:

Affirmations about the recovery journey:

9

Women's Empowerment and Recovery-Oriented Care

A New Intervention Model

As we have discussed in the previous chapters, women with serious mental illness (SMI) commonly seek mental health services. However, the specific needs and experiences of these women are often overlooked in treatment and research. To fill this gap in research and care, we created the *Women's Empowerment and Recovery-Oriented Care* (WE-ROC) intervention. WE-ROC is a manualized group that integrates recovery-oriented and feminist approaches into mental health care in order to boost participants' mental wellness and empowerment. In this final chapter, we will review the treatment research on women with SMI and, based on this, present our new model for integrating gender-sensitive therapy and recovery-oriented care for women with SMI. We will present data suggesting the promise of this group intervention from a pilot study. In addition, we will discuss other clinical applications of this model and future directions for research and clinical work with women with SMI.

TREATMENT RESEARCH ON WOMEN WITH SMI

A review of the literature suggested the need for a new mental health intervention for women with SMI. To the best of our knowledge, no interventions have been published that more generally target the issues of women with SMI to date. Much of the identifiable research in this area has focused on maternal mental health. For example, a systematic review (Doucet, Jones, Letourneau, Dennis, & Blackmore, 2011) found 26 studies on postpartum psychosis from 1973 through 2008, including both treatment and prevention studies. Other intervention studies include an antenatal group for pregnant women with depression and anxiety (Thomas, Komiti, & Judd, 2014) and a dialectical behavior therapy group for perinatal adolescents with depression (Kleiber et al., 2017). It appears that much of the treatment innovation in this area has focused on reducing the risks surrounding motherhood for women with SMI.

A few intervention studies have been conducted that pertain to other aspects of the lives of women with SMI. For instance, there is the Seeking Safety intervention for people with dual-diagnosis substance abuse and other mental health problems. This cognitive-behavioral therapy manualized intervention was evaluated in an open trial design with a population of mostly incarcerated women with SMI as well as post-traumatic stress disorder (PTSD) and substance use disorder (Wolff, Frueh, Shi, & Schumann, 2012). Another study involved evaluating the Seeking Safety intervention (Cusack, Morrisey, & Ellis, 2008). The researchers found that it was most effective for women with high levels of PTSD rather than those with few symptoms. Again, these interventions have focused more on issues of risk among women with SMI.

Other relevant intervention research has had a broader focus in terms of population, including women with mental health problems but without SMI. For example, a randomized controlled trial was conducted of a CBT group for women with depression (Cramer, Salisbury, Conrad, Eldred, & Araya, 2011). Another pilot study (Collins, Geller, Miller, Toro, & Susser, 2001) involved a 10-module protocol developed for women with SMI. This pilot included psychoeducation and behavioral training to reduce the risk of contracting and transmitting HIV. These groups have brought an important focus on maternal mental health, substance abuse, PTSD, depression, incarceration, or HIV prevention. However, no identifiable studies have featured the development and evaluation of an intervention that addresses both the specific and wide-ranging needs of women with SMI.

A conceptual framework for the present intervention with women with SMI was developed in a larger qualitative study with selective investigation in several key areas. These central issues pertained to the following: dating and relationships (Mizock, LaMar, DeMartini, & Stringer, 2019), treatment by family and providers (Mizock & Brubaker, in press), challenges with work and financial wellness (Mizock, Aitken, & LaMar, 2019) and the benefits of affirming the unique strengths of women with SMI (Lloyd & Mizock, 2018). This led to the development of several modules (Table 9.1) that we will discuss here.

INTERVENTION FRAMEWORK

WE-ROC was created to address the needs of women with SMI using recovery-oriented care and feminist therapy principles. Some of the largest mental health associations have emphasized the need for recovery-oriented care for people with SMI, including the Substance Abuse and Mental Health Services Administration (SAMHSA), the Institute of Medicine, the American Psychological Association (APA & Jansen, 2014), and the U.S. Surgeon General (SAMHSA, 2015). As discussed in Chapter 3, the term "recovery" is borrowed from the substance abuse field. In the context of a mental illness, recovery does not refer to symptom elimination alone; rather, recovery entails seeking a life of hope, meaning, and

Table 9.1 WE-ROC content overview

Treatment Session	Treatment Elements
Week #1 Introduction to WE-ROC	• <u>Baseline Assessment</u>: Complete paperwork, including baseline assessments of empowerment and recovery scores • <u>Introduction</u>: Group facilitators and members introduce themselves • <u>Overview</u>: Review group model and group schedule • <u>Activity</u>: Ground rules and member group goals • <u>Didactics</u>: Concepts of recovery and empowerment • <u>Homework</u>: Introduce and assign "Power Tool" coping strategy
Week #2 Gender, Recovery, and Stigma	• <u>Introduction</u>: Check-in, review ground rules, last session summary, discuss "Power Tool" coping strategy from past week • <u>Didactics</u>: Concepts of stigma, self-stigma, and double stigma • <u>Discussion</u>: Experiences with mental health and gender stigma • <u>Activity</u>: Empowered woman visualization • <u>Homework</u>: Assign "Power Tool" coping strategy
Week #3 Family, Dating, and Relationships	• <u>Introduction</u>: Check-in, review ground rules, last session summary, discuss "Power Tool" coping strategy from past week • <u>Didactics</u>: Research on the experiences of women with SMI in family, dating, and relationships • <u>Discussion</u>: Experiences with family, dating, and relationships • <u>Activity</u>: Relationship goals • <u>Homework</u>: Assign "Power Tool" coping strategy
Week #4 Experiences with Mental Health Care	• <u>Introduction</u>: Check-in, review ground rules, last session summary, discuss "Power Tool" coping strategy from past week • <u>Discussion</u>: Experiences with mental health care • <u>Didactics</u>: Principles of recovery-oriented and empowering care • <u>Activity</u>: Inner therapist visualization • <u>Homework</u>: Assign "Power Tool" coping strategy
Week #5 Meaningful Work and Financial Wellness	• <u>Introduction</u>: Check-in, review ground rules, last session summary, discuss "Power Tool" coping strategy from past week • <u>Didactics</u>: Research on women with SMI, work, and money • <u>Discussion</u>: Experiences with work and money • <u>Activity</u>: In pairs, identify strengths and goals in work and money • <u>Homework</u>: Assign "Power Tool" coping strategy

(*continued*)

Table 9.1 CONTINUED

Treatment Session	Treatment Elements
Week #6 Affirming Strengths	• Introduction: Check-in, review ground rules, last session summary, discuss "Power Tool" coping strategy from past week • Discussion: Gender and mental health strengths as woman • Didactics: Concepts of resilience and self-esteem • Activity: Inspiring quote card for personal affirmation • Homework: Assign "Power Tool" coping strategy and Community Action Project ideas
Week #7 Community Action and Empowerment	• Introduction: Check-in, review ground rules, last session summary, discuss "Power Tool" coping strategy from past week • Didactics: Concept of community action • Discussion: Discuss and identify community action needed for women with mental health challenges • Activity: Plan and possibly carry out community action activity. Plan final group celebration and reflection meeting. • Homework: Assign "Power Tool" coping strategy
Week #8 Group Reflection and Celebration	• Introduction: Check-in, review ground rules, last session summary, discuss "Power Tool" coping strategy from past week, distribute and review "Power Tools" created by group • Discussion: Reflect on experience of group and ending • Activity: Group member affirmation activity and time for celebration

From Mizock (2019). Reprinted with permission from *Psychiatric Rehabilitation Journal* © 2019.

self-determination and not being defined by one's mental illness. Recovery-oriented care for people with SMI incorporates values of psychiatric rehabilitation, which focuses on boosting functioning to support their ability to participate in daily life across daily contexts. The approach is person-centered and collaborative, focused on the individual's preferences, goals, and growth potential, regardless of challenges (Anthony & Farkas, 2009). In this model, rehabilitation is viewed as possible without symptom reduction, and role functioning is considered just as important as symptom eradication.

WE-ROC also integrates the principles of feminist therapy in order to raise awareness of gender issues to boost empowerment. Conlin (2017) provided a review of feminist therapy, noting several tenets that have demonstrated empirical support in achieving therapy outcomes. Some primary goals of feminist therapy are empowerment, agency, and enhanced coping of the client in reaction to sources of oppression as they impact mental health, rather than a traditional focus on alleviating symptoms. This therapy also builds a collaborative relationship between the therapist and client, with attention to how power is enacted in the therapeutic alliance and other relationships in the client's life. Consciousness raising is used to enhance the client's awareness about the effects of oppression on psychological distress, increasing self-esteem and self-efficacy. These elements of feminist therapy are present within the WE-ROC philosophical framework. As discussed in Chapter 1, feminist therapy has come to be referred to in some cases as "gender-sensitive" therapy in order to be inclusive beyond just the female gender (Walker, 2009). Hence, we use "gender-sensitive therapy" to refer to feminist clinical practice.

Eight treatment modules of WE-ROC were developed (see Table 9.1) to focus on issues of recovery and empowerment. These modules were developed from our aforementioned research, the extant literature, and the recovery and feminist principles we just described. Discussion and didactic segments were conducted to enhance awareness of the impact of gender on mental health and to provide group support for collective experiences surrounding the experience of women with SMI. Topics of family, dating, and relationships were addressed. Positive and negative experiences in mental health care were explored, as well as strategies to advocate for one's care. Experiences with meaningful work and financial challenges were also covered, given the employment barriers and financial issues facing this group. The women in the group were supported to identify their strengths pertaining to their gender and mental health identities in order to boost their self-esteem. Finally, the group engaged in community action through structured activities. This created a sense of agency and empowerment in working toward the social change that women with SMI desire in their communities.

THE PILOT STUDY

The pilot of the WE-ROC intervention included 10 women with SMI. Specific information on the participants, methodology, and results is given in the publication on this topic (Mizock, 2019). To summarize, all participants were 18 years of age and older; had a diagnosis of an SMI (bipolar disorder, severe depression, or schizophrenia); and reported major impairment in functioning in occupational, social, and activities of daily living.

The WE-ROC intervention was conducted for eight sessions, meeting once a week for a 1.5- to 2-hour session. The group was facilitated by a peer specialist who is a woman with the lived experience of an SMI. Participants completed pretest and posttest measures to assess the effectiveness of the intervention as part of the pre-experimental, pretest–posttest, repeated-measures design.

The WE-ROC curriculum includes structured discussions, experiential exercises, skills teaching, and community action activities (see Table 9.1). Each group began with an introduction, including a review of ground rules, check-in, a summary of the previous group, and a discussion of the out-of-session assignment from the previous week. This section was typically followed by structured discussions, didactic content pertaining to several key concepts for the day, and experiential exercises/activities. At the end of each session, an out-of-session task was assigned based on the topic of that day.

There are a number of recovery assessment measures that can be useful for measuring recovery in people with SMI. Several of these measures were used to assess pre–post changes in recovery and empowerment and to elicit participant feedback. The first measure is the *Recovery Assessment Scale* (RAS; see Corrigan, Salzer, Ralph, Sangster, & Keck, 2004). The RAS was used to assess pretest–posttest changes in recovery scores. The 41 items are rated using a 5-point Likert scale (1 = strongly disagree; 5 = strongly agree). This scale assesses recovery levels, including goals, knowledge of symptom management, and ability to cope. For example, one item on the scale reads: "I can identify what triggers the symptoms of my mental illness."

The *Empowerment Scale* (see Rogers, Chamberlin, Ellison, & Crean, 1997) for users of mental health services was also used to assess pretest–posttest changes in empowerment. The 28 items are rated using on a 4-point Likert scale (1 = strongly disagree; 4 = strongly agree). The scale assesses empowerment levels, including locus of control, attitude toward recovery, and self-worth. An example of an item on the scale is: "I avoid people on the street whose gender is unclear to me."

The *Participant Feedback Inventory*, a flexible mixed-methods scale that is partly quantitative and partly qualitative, was developed for the WE-ROC intervention to gather feedback tailored to the intervention. Statistical reliability analysis and content analysis were conducted on this form to refine the inventory. This revised version is included at the end of this chapter. This inventory might hold utility for future WE-ROC interventions, or for evaluating other therapy groups.

The survey data were analyzed using descriptive and inferential statistical analyses. Content analysis was conducted to identify categories of feedback provided on the open-ended section of the feedback form and to quantify the frequency of different types of feedback using multiple coders. Feedback was quantified per conceptual content analysis in order to arrive at frequencies of categories of feedback.

The details of the results of the study have been published elsewhere (Mizock, 2019). In sum, the findings suggest that the intervention was assessed to have strong feasibility and to hold promise for boosting recovery and empowerment among women with SMI. The feasibility of the intervention was reflected by the high attendance rates. Its acceptability was indicated in the high intervention satisfaction scores and effectiveness scores. Exploratory correlational analysis found an association between empowerment and recovery scores, suggesting that higher recovery scores were associated with higher empowerment scores. Correlational analysis also suggested that as the weeks progressed, participants generally rated the interventions with increasingly higher levels of satisfaction and effectiveness. This finding suggests that the building of group cohesion over the course of the group could lead the participants to find the group more satisfying and effective in its aims.

Content analysis of the qualitative feedback revealed that one of the greatest gains of this group was connecting with peers, as might be expected in a group format. Participants also frequently reported that they had learned from the group via the didactic content presented. They also reported boosts in self-esteem, which, anecdotally, was a common personal goal set by participants at the onset of the group. While these women appeared to enjoy many of the activities, they also had a number of suggestions for various modifications. There were requests for stronger facilitation and clarity about the content, which are planned to be addressed in future iterations of the intervention.

The results supported the use of the RAS and the Empowerment Scale to evaluate pre–post recovery and empowerment scores in future studies of the intervention. In addition, the revised feedback form used in the pilot also appears to hold promise as a flexible measure for pre–post mixed-methods evaluation on new interventions. Reliability data were somewhat weak at times, leading to the aforementioned revision of the form as it appears at the end of this chapter.

The WE-ROC pilot was a pre-experimental study, and future research on this intervention would benefit from a number of research conditions. A waitlist control group could help to determine if changes in baseline occurred as an artifact of time. Additional assessment at six months after the intervention could also be included to evaluate for longer-term benefits of the group. A larger sample size could also boost statistical power. It should also be noted that the group was predominantly White and East Asian American, as well as heterosexual. Furthermore, the group was mostly made up of women with diagnoses of bipolar disorder and severe depression rather than schizophrenia spectrum diagnoses. Future waves of the intervention could have more diversity, particularly with regard to racial-ethnic background, diagnosis, and sexual orientation. It would also be important to enhance empowerment scores across age groups in further testing, given that age was found to co-vary with empowerment. Overall, the intervention holds considerable promise for future iterations and could be refined with a number of revisions based on participant feedback.

APPLICATIONS TO CLINICAL WORK

The WE-ROC intervention reflects the feminist therapy and recovery-oriented principles of our psychotherapy model. Our model holds applications to other areas of clinical work with people with SMI. We will discuss a few relevant applications here.

To start, WE-ROC's development and evaluation reflect the inherent value of egalitarian therapy relationships. This is a foundational construct of feminist therapy and recovery-oriented care. Relationship building is central to the recovery journey (Spaniol et al., 2002). The relationships formed between group participants and the peer facilitator provided a context for building empowerment, coping strategies, and daily living skills. In fact, participant responses indicated that one of the most valuable aspects of the WE-ROC intervention was being able to connect with other women with SMI in this context.

The WE-ROC intervention holds insights for systems of care in fostering the recovery journey of individuals. Traditional models tend to relegate consumers to the "patient" role and overlook their uniquely gendered experiences, without engaging them as experts in their care (Manuel, Hinterland, Conover, & Herman, 2012; Slade, 2009). The WE-ROC model can support therapeutic relationships in which individuals are valued for their strengths and capabilities and can also provide a forum for self-direction and empowerment. Women and men with SMI can be seen as experts in their own mental health experiences, and gender can be understood as a core component of their recovery.

The WE-ROC intervention also provides value for the use of peer specialists in providing recovery-oriented and gender-responsive interventions. Peer specialists can be used in mental health treatment to demonstrate an egalitarian stance in the group facilitation, drawing from the lived experience of a person with a mental health problem. The use of peer support has been found to have a positive impact in many ways, such as increasing quality of life, empowerment, and levels of hope (Bellamy, Schmutte, & Davidson, 2017). This current study adds to that literature through the use of a peer specialist to facilitate the group.

Finally, WE-ROC can be adapted for use with men. The authors are working on future projects to develop a ME-ROC (Men's Empowerment and Recovery-Oriented Care) group intervention. Some of the group components of WE-ROC would be used in ME-ROC, while others would be quite different. Other content might cover the gender socialization of men in traditional masculinity, which idealizes White, wealthy, muscular, and educated men (Courtenay, 2000). Per this model, men are conditioned to take greater health risks and to avoid seeking help. The ME-ROC intervention would discuss the experience of men with SMI with these cultural messages and the implications for their recovery.

CONCLUSION

The WE-ROC manualized group intervention offers an exciting new format for the delivery of care for women with SMI. Future directions include conducting additional waves of this group with different samples, and adapting this intervention to provide a gender-sensitive and recovery-oriented care intervention for men. It is our hope that this book can inspire other treatment innovations that address the needs of women, men, and gender nonbinary people with SMI in a gender-sensitive manner to boost their empowerment, recovery, and agency.

CLINICAL STRATEGIES LIST

- Explore with women with SMI the intersections of sexism, stigma, and other types of oppression. Discuss how they cope with these experiences and overcome them. Empower women to identify the strengths that have helped them to face their challenges. Help them identify how they can continue to use those strengths to address their current challenges.

- Validate and name women's experiences of gender and mental health oppression. This process can foster alliance building and the safety to call out experiences of discrimination for what they are. Encourage women with SMI to be bold in speaking out about these issues.
- Discuss the impact of stigma and its effects on women's mental health. Instill hope in the capacity of women with SMI to recover.
- Help women with SMI to identify the resources they have and ones they would like to develop. Advocate for their pursuit of goals that fit within their vision of recovery, whether it be financial independence, stable housing, or belonging to a particular community.
- Find out what a woman with SMI believes her providers need to learn about her to effectively partner with her. Ask her to identify what she would like to teach new medical students, psychology fellows, and new nursing staff in this area. If possible, provide opportunities for the woman to share this with her treatment team. See if she would like to join in efforts to teach new trainees or new staff at your organization. This could involve speaking on a panel at a new staff or trainee orientation. It might be empowering for these women to share their knowledge to benefit the care of others.
- Help women with SMI to identify activism they might be interested in taking part in. This might include advocating for more state or federal funds to be allocated to housing, supported employment, or mental health services. Women with SMI might also be encouraged to advocate within their mental health system to transform service provision. This could include eliminating coercive or punitive practices, or serving as peer advocates in the involuntary hospitalization process. There, they could help other people with SMI to understand their rights or engage in other advocacy efforts.

DISCUSSION QUESTIONS

The following discussion questions are adapted from the WE-ROC intervention:

1. What are your experiences with gender-related stigma or sexism as a person of your gender? Are there any ways in which things are different for women with mental health problems than for men or gender diverse people? Have you internalized any of this stigma, leading to self-stigma? What do your experiences tell you about what this might be like for people with SMI?
2. How might relationships be impacted for women with SMI? Specifically consider dating, friendship, parenting, and family relationships. What about for men or gender nonbinary people? Are there similarities

or differences? How might mental health providers support them in pursuing their relationship goals and challenging mistreatment in relationships?

3. What are some of the implications and applications of gender-sensitive and recovery-oriented care for men with SMI? For transgender and gender nonbinary people? What might future group interventions for these populations look like?

ACTIVITIES

The following activities are adapted from the WE-ROC intervention:

1. Empowered Woman Visualization. Prepare yourself for a creative visualization activity that is adapted from Tara Mohr (2015). You will paint a picture in your mind. If you have trouble imagining things in your mind, you can write about what you might envision or draw a picture. Take a few deep breaths and get relaxed in your chair. Imagine yourself as strong and empowered. What do you see yourself doing? How do you feel? What are your thoughts like? Who is around you? After completing this exercise, draw or journal about this empowering vision of yourself in the future when you want to connect to a vision of your own strength. How did the experience feel? What might be the benefits to conducting this visualization with women and men with SMI? What are the implications for issues of gender and empowerment? How might you conduct this visualization with a group of people with SMI?

2. Power Tool. The WE-ROC intervention involves identifying empowering coping strategies to practice each week (also known as a "Power Tool"). List your power tools for managing stress and create a handout (perhaps collapsing with those of others in a group) to disseminate to others.

3. Community Action. Identify one small step toward taking community action for women with mental health challenges, and carry this out. This might include making cards to support women who are in shelters or have mental health challenges, writing to news media sources requesting coverage of issues for women with mental health challenges, volunteering, writing a letter to a congressperson, fundraising, donating, mentoring someone, joining a group, starting a petition online or signing one, learning about political candidates in an election and voting, challenging stigma in popular culture, or educating someone you know about mental health issues. What was it like for you to take this action? How might people with SMI experience this activity? Based on your experience, reflect on some barriers that people with SMI might face in carrying out community action. What might help them to do it to enhance a sense of empowerment?

PARTICIPANT FEEDBACK INVENTORY

1. Please provide feedback on your experience of these parts of the group:

    Satisfaction? (10 = Very Satisfied)

    a) Topics discussed   Score (1–10) _____

    b) Activities   Score (1–10) _____

    c) Facilitation   Score (1–10) _____

    d) Group members   Score (1–10) _____

    e) Impact on self-esteem/mental health Score (1–10) _____

    f) Overall group satisfaction   Score (1–10) _____

    g) Other (write in:) _____ Score (1–10) _____(or N/A)

2. Please explain any feedback above or provide other feedback you have about the group today:

    _____

    _____

    _____

Lauren Mizock, PhD, is Core Faculty in the Clinical Psychology Ph.D. program at Fielding Graduate University and Director of the Social Justice and Diversity Concentration. Dr. Mizock published the books *Acceptance of Mental Illness: Promoting Recovery Among Culturally Diverse Groups* (Oxford University Press, 2016) and *Researcher Race: Social Constructions in the Research Process* (Information Age Publishing, 2012), in addition to over 60 publications. Dr. Mizock is on the Executive Committee of the Society for the Psychology of Women (Division 35) of the American Psychological Association (APA) and co-chairs, with Dr. Carr, the Women with Serious Mental Illness Committee and Motherhood Committee. Dr. Mizock co-edited a special issue of the journal of *Women & Therapy*, "Women with Serious Mental Illness in Therapy: Intersectional Perspectives" (2015). Dr. Mizock is a licensed clinical psychologist and maintains a private practice in San Francisco. She is the recipient of several awards and grants related to mental health, diversity, and public service, including the Early Career Diversity Award and Psychotherapy with Women Awards from the APA. Dr. Mizock's research and clinical interests are in cultural competence in teaching and clinical practice, serious mental illness, women's mental health, and transgender and gender-diverse populations. In her spare time, Dr. Mizock enjoys yoga, the beach, museums, and other city adventures with her husband and toddler near their home in San Francisco.

Erika Carr, PhD, is in a tenure-track position as an Assistant Professor in the Department of Psychiatry at Yale University School of Medicine and also serves as Director of the Inpatient Psychology Service at Connecticut Mental Health Center in New Haven, CT. Dr. Carr is the Chair of the Task Force for Women Who Experience Serious Mental Illness in the Society for the Psychology of Women (Division 35) of the American Psychological Association (APA). Dr. Carr is also a licensed psychologist in New Haven, CT. Dr. Carr was awarded the Psychotherapy with Women Award in August 2013 from Division 35, Psychology of Women of APA. Dr. Carr provides clinical care with individuals who experience serious mental illness and has a particular interest in women who experience serious mental illness, as evident by her focus on women's issues and recovery-oriented care. Dr. Carr directs the psychology service at her institution for an inpatient psychiatric unit and specifically focuses on providing training experiences for psychology fellows from a recovery-oriented perspective so as to help empower the individuals they serve, mitigating the impact of stigma and oppression, and partnering in the recovery journeys of individuals who experience serious mental illness as they build lives of meaning as they so define.

BIBLIOGRAPHY

Abernethy, A. D., Houston, T. R., Mimms, T., & Boyd-Franklin, N. (2006). Using prayer in psychotherapy: Applying Sue's differential to enhance culturally competent care. *Cultural Diversity & Ethnic Minority Psychology, 12*, 101–114.

Ackerson, B. J. (2003). Coping with the dual demands of severe mental illness and parenting: The parents' perspective. *Families in Society, 84*(1), 109–118.

Adams, N., & Grieder, D. M. (2013). *Treatment planning for person-centered care: Shared-decision making for whole health.* New York, NY: Academic Press.

Adler, N. E., Epel, E. S., Castellazo, G., & Ickovics, J. R. (2000). Relationship of subjective and objective social status with psychological and physiological functioning: Preliminary data in healthy white women. *Health Psychology, 19*(6), 586–592.

Akutsu, P. D., Snowden, L. R., & Organista, K. C. (1996). Referral patterns in ethnic-specific and mainstream programs for ethnic minorities and whites. *Journal of Counseling Psychology, 43*, 56–64.

Albers, D. A. (1973). Involuntary hospitalization: Observations on the politics of a coalition. *South Dakota Law Review, 18*, 348.

Alegría, M., Canino, G., Shrout, P. E., Woo, M., Duan, N., . . . Meng, X. (2008). Prevalence of mental illness in immigrant and non-immigrant groups. *American Journal of Psychiatry, 165*, 359–369.

Allison, D. B., Mentore, J. L., Heo, M., Chandler, L. P., Cappelleri, J. C., Infante, M. C., & Weiden, P. J. (1999). Antipsychotic-induced weight gain: A comprehensive research synthesis. *American Journal of Psychiatry, 156*, 1686–1696.

Altamura, A. C., Sassella, F., Santini, A., Montresor, C., Fumagalli, S., & Mundo, E. (2003). Intramuscular preparations of antipsychotics: Uses and relevance in clinical practice. *Drugs, 63*, 493–512.

Alverson, H. S., Drake, R. E., Carpenter-Song, E. A., Chu, E., Ritsema, M., & Smith, B. (2007). Ethnocultural variations in mental illness discourse: Some implications for building therapeutic alliances. *Psychiatric Services, 58*(12), 1541–1546.

American Academy of Pediatrics Committee on Drugs. (2000). Use of psychoactive medication during pregnancy and possible effects on the fetus and newborn. *Pediatrics, 105*, 880–887.

American Psychiatric Association. (2010). Mental health disparities: American Indians and Alaska Natives. APA Fact Sheet. Retrieved from https://www.integration. samhsa.gov/workforce/mental_health_disparities_american_indian_and_alaskan_ natives.pdf

American Psychiatric Association. (2013). *Diagnostic and statistical manual of mental disorders* (5th ed.). Washington, DC: American Psychiatric Association.

American Psychological Association & Jansen, M. (2014). *Reframing psychology for the emerging health care environment: Recovery curriculum for people with serious mental illnesses and behavioral health disorders.* Washington, DC: American Psychological Association.

Anderson, A. (2014). Childless by choice: Parenting and mental illness. *The Toast.* Retrieved from http://the-toast.net/2014/04/07having-no-children-and-having-mental-illness/

Andrews, H. B. (2001). Back to basics: Psychotherapy is an interpersonal process. *Australian Psychologist, 36*(2), 107–114.

Anthony, M., & Berg, M. J. (2002a). Biologic and molecular mechanisms for sex differences in pharmacokinetics, pharmacodynamics, and pharmacogenetics, part I. *Journal of Women's Health and Gender-Based Medicine, 11*, 601–615.

Anthony, M., & Berg, M. J. (2002b). Biologic and molecular mechanisms for sex differences in pharmacokinetics, pharmacodynamics, and pharmacogenetics, part II. *Journal of Women's Health and Gender-Based Medicine, 11*, 617–629.

Anthony, W. (1993). Recovery from mental illness: The guiding vision of the mental health service system in the 1990s. *Psychosocial Rehabilitation Journal, 16*, 11–23.

Anthony, W. A., & Farkas, M. D. (2009). *Primer on the psychiatric rehabilitation process.* Boston, MA: University Center for Psychiatric Rehabilitation.

Armour, M. P., Bradshaw, W., & Roseborough, D. (2009). African Americans and recovery from severe mental illness. *Social Work in Mental Health, 7*(6), 602–622.

Artazcoz, L., Benach, J., Borrell, C., & Cortès, I. (2004). Unemployment and mental health: Understanding the interactions among gender, family roles, and social class. *American Journal of Public Health, 94*(1), 82–88.

Ashcraft, L., Bloss, M., & Anthony, W. A. (2012). Best practices: The development and implementation of "no force first" as a best practice. *Psychiatric Services, 63*(5), 415–417.

Bach, P., Gaudiano, B. A., Hayes, S. C., & Herbert, J. D. (2013). Acceptance and commitment therapy for psychosis: Intent to treat, hospitalization outcome and mediation by believability. *Psychosis, 5*(2), 166–174.

Balant-Gorgia, A. E., Gex-Fabry, M., & Balant, L. P. (1996). Therapeutic drug monitoring and drug–drug interactions: A pharmacoepidemiological perspective. *Therapy, 51*, 399–402.

Barber, M. E. (2009). Lesbian, gay, and bisexual people with severe mental illness. *Journal of Gay & Lesbian Mental Health, 13*(2), 133–142.

Beck, J. C., & van der Kolk, B. (1987). Reports of childhood incest and current behavior of chronically hospitalized psychotic women. *American Journal of Psychiatry, 144*, 1474–1476.

Becker, D., Liver, O., Mester, R., Rapoport, M., Weizman, A., & Weiss, M. (2003). Risperdone, but not olanzapine, decreases bone mineral density in female premenopausal schizophrenia patients. *Journal of Clinical Psychiatry, 64*, 761–766.

Beierle, I., Meibohm, B., & Derendorf, H. (1999). Gender differences in pharmacokinetics and pharmacodynamics. *International Journal of Clinical Pharmacological Therapy, 37*, 529–647.

Beiser, M., Bean, G., Erickson, D., Zhang, J., Iacono, W. G., & Rector, N. A. (1994). Biological and psychosocial predictors of job performance following a first episode of psychosis. *American Journal of Psychiatry, 151*, 857–863.

Bellack, A. S., Mueser, K. T., Gingerich, S., & Agresta, J. (2013). *Social skills training for schizophrenia: A step-by-step guide.* New York, NY: Guilford Publications.

Bellamy, C., Schmutte, T., & Davidson, L. (2017). An update on the growing evidence base for peer support. *Mental Health and Social Inclusion, 21*(3), 161–167.

Belle, D. (1990). Poverty and women's mental health. *American Psychologist, 45*(3), 385–389.

Benbow, S., Forchuk, C., & Ray, S. L. (2011). Mothers with mental illness experiencing homelessness: A critical analysis. *Journal of Psychiatric and Mental Health Nursing, 18,* 687–695.

Bergström, T., Seikkula, J., Alakare, B., Mäki, P., Köngäs-Saviaro, P., Taskila, J. J., . . . Aaltonen, J. (2018). The family-oriented open dialogue approach in the treatment of first-episode psychosis: Nineteen-year outcomes. *Psychiatry Research, 270,* 168–175.

Bhugra, D. (2006). Severe mental illness across cultures. *Acta Psychiatria Scandinavica, 113*(Suppl. 429), 17–23.

Bildt, C., & Michelsen, H. (2002). Gender differences in the effects from working conditions on mental health: A 4-year follow-up. *International Archives of Occupational and Environmental Health, 75,* 252–258.

Bloom, S. L. (1997). *Creating sanctuary: Toward the evolution of sane societies.* New York, NY: Routledge.

Boyle, R. J. (2002). Effects of certain prenatal drugs on the fetus and newborn. *Pediatric Review, 23,* 17–24.

Braslow, J. T. (1996). In the name of therapeutics: The practice of sterilization in a California State Hospital. *Journal of the History of Medicine and Allied Sciences, 51,* 29–51.

Braslow, J. T., & Starks, S. L. (2005). The making of contemporary American psychiatry, part 2: Therapeutics and gender before and after World War II. *History of Psychology, 8*(3), 271–288.

Breier, A., & Strauss, J. S. (1984). The role of social relationships in the recovery from psychotic disorders. *American Journal of Psychiatry, 141,* 949–955.

Breslau, N., Chilcoat, H. D., Kessler, R. C., Peterson, E. L., & Lucia, V. C. (1999). Vulnerability to assaultive violence: Further specification of the sex difference in post-traumatic stress disorder. *Psychological Medicine, 29,* 813–821.

Breslau, N., Kessler, R. C., Chilcoat, H. D., Schultz, L. R., Davis, G. C., & Andreski, P. (1998). Trauma and posttraumatic stress disorder in the community: The 1996 Detroit Area Survey of Trauma. *Archives of General Psychiatry, 55,* 626–632.

Briggs, M. K., & Dixon, A. L. (2013). Women's spirituality across the life span: Implications for counseling. *Counseling and Values, 58*(1), 104–120.

Brown, L. (2009). Cultural competence: A new way of thinking about integration in therapy. *Journal of Psychotherapy Integration, 19*(4), 340–353.

Brown, S., Birtwistle, J., Roe, L., & Thompson, C. (1999). The unhealthy lifestyle of people with schizophrenia. *Psychological Medicine, 29,* 697–701.

Buchanan, T. S., Fischer, A. R., Tokar, D. M., & Yoder, J. D. (2008). Testing a culture-specific extension of objectification theory regarding African American women's body image. *Counseling Psychologist, 36,* 699–718.

Buckley, P. F., Robben, T., Friedman, L., & Hyde, J. (1999). Sexual behavior in persons with serious mental illness: Patterns and clinical correlates. In P. F. Buckley

(Ed.), *Sexuality and serious mental illness* (pp. 1–21). Amsterdam: Harwood Academic Press.

Burke, J. G., Gielen, A. C., McDonnell, K. A., O'Campo, P., & Maman, S. (2001). The process of ending abuse in intimate relationships: A qualitative exploration of the transtheoretical model. *Violence Against Women, 7*(10), 1144–1163.

Burney, J., & Irwin, H. J. (2000). Shame and guilt in women with eating-disorder symptomatology. *Journal of Clinical Psychology, 56,* 51–61.

Calogero, R. M. (2004). A test of objectification theory: The effect of the male gaze on appearance concerns in college women. *Psychology of Women Quarterly, 28,* 16–21.

Calogero, R. M., & Jost, J. T. (2011). Self-subjugation among women: Exposure to sexist ideology, self-objectification, and the protective function of the need to avoid closure. *Journal of Personality and Social Psychology, 100*(2), 211.

Campbell, J. C. (2002). Safety planning based on lethality assessment for partners of batterers in intervention programs. *Journal of Aggression, Maltreatment, and Trauma, 5*(2), 129–143.

Campbell, J. C. (2004). Helping women understand their risk in situations of intimate partner violence. *Journal of Interpersonal Violence, 19*(12), 1464–1477.

Carey, M. P., Carey, K. B., Maisto, S. A., Gordon, C. M., & Vanable, P. A. (2001). Prevalence and correlates of sexual activity and HIV-related risk behavior among psychiatric outpatients. *Journal of Consulting and Clinical Psychology, 69,* 846–50.

Carmen, E. H., Rieker, P. P., & Mills, T. (1987). *Victims of violence and psychiatric illness.* Washington, DC: American Psychiatric Press.

Carpenter, W. T., & Kirkpatrick, B. (1988). The heterogeneity of the long-term outcome of schizophrenia. *Schizophrenia Bulletin, 14,* 645–652.

Carpenter-Song, E., Chu, E., Drake, R. E., Ritsema, M., Smith, B., & Alverson, H. (2010). Ethno-cultural variations in the experience and meaning of mental illness and treatment: Implications for access and utilization. *Transcultural Psychiatry, 47*(2), 224–251.

Carpenter-Song, E., Whitley, R., Lawson, W., Quimby, E., & Drake, R. E. (2011). Reducing disparities in mental health care: Suggestions from the Dartmouth-Howard collaboration. *Community Mental Health Journal, 47,* 1–13.

Carr, E., Greene, B., & Ponce, A. (2015). Women and the experience of serious mental illness and sexual objectification: Multicultural feminist theoretical frameworks and therapy recommendations. *Women and Therapy, 38*(1/2), 53–76.

Carr, E., & Szymanski, D. M. (2011). Sexual objectification and substance abuse in young adult women. *Counseling Psychologist, 39,* 39–66.

Carter, R. T. (2007). Racism and psychological and emotional injury: Recognizing and assessing race-based traumatic stress. *Counseling Psychologist, 35*(13), 73–96.

Cascardi, M., Mueser, K. T., DeGiralomo, J., & Murrin, M. (1996). Physical aggression against psychiatric inpatients by family members and partners. *Psychiatric Services, 47,* 531–533.

Casey, D. (1991). Neuroleptic drug-induced extrapyramidal syndromes and tardive dyskinesia. *Schizophrenia Research, 4,* 109–120.

Casper, R. (2008). *Women's health: Hormones, emotions and behavior.* Palo Alto, CA: Stanford University.

Cervantes, J. M. (2010). Mestizo spirituality: Toward an integrated approach to psychotherapy for Latinas/os. *Psychotherapy Theory: Research, Practice, Training, 47*(4), 527–539.

Chandy, J. M., Blum, R. W. M., & Resnick, M. D. (1996). Gender-specific outcomes for sexually abused adolescents. *Child Abuse & Neglect, 20*, 1319–1331.

Chang, C. K., Hayes, R. D., Perera, G., Broadbent, M. T., Fernandes, A. C., Lee, W. E., . . . Stewart, R. (2011). Life expectancy at birth for people with serious mental illness and other major disorders from a secondary mental health care case register in London. *PLoS One, 6*, e19590.

Chen, S. X., & Mak, W. S. (2008). Seeking professional help: Etiology beliefs about mental illness across cultures. *Journal of Counseling Psychology, 55*(4), 442–450.

Chernomas, W. M., Clarke, D. E., & Chisholm, F. A. (2000). The perspectives of women living with serious mental illness. *Psychiatric Services, 51*(12), 1517–1521.

Chesler, P. (2005). *Women and madness*. New York, NY: Palgrave MacMillan.

Clements-Nolle, K., Marx, R., & Katz, M. (2006). Attempted suicide among transgender persons. *Journal of Homosexuality, 51*(3), 53–69.

Cook, J. (2000). Sexuality and people with disabilities. *Sexuality and Disability, 18*(3), 195–206.

Collins, P. Y., Geller, P. A., Miller, S., Toro, P., & Susser, E. S. (2001). Ourselves, our bodies, our realities: An HIV prevention intervention for women with severe mental illness. *Journal of Urban Health: Bulletin of the New York Academy of Medicine, 78*(1), 162–175.

Collins, P. Y., Sweetland, A., & Zybert, P. (2007). *How dangerous is stigma? Stigma and HIV risk among women with severe mental illness*. Presented at the 160th Annual Meeting of the American Psychiatric Association, San Diego, CA.

Collins, P. Y., von Unger, H., & Ambrister, A. (2008). Church ladies, good girls, and locas: Stigma and the intersection of gender, ethnicity, mental illness, and sexuality in relation to HIV risk. *Social Science & Medicine, 67*, 389–397.

Colton, C. W., & Manderscheid, R. W. (2006). Congruencies in increased mortality rates, years of potential life lost, and causes of death among public mental health clients in eight states. *Prevention of Chronic Disease, 3*, A42.

Condino, V., Tanzilli, A., Speranza, A. M., & Lingiardi, V. (2016). Therapeutic interventions in intimate partner violence: An overview. *Research in Psychotherapy: Psychopathology, Process and Outcome, 19*(2).

Conlin, S. E. (2017). Feminist therapy: A brief integrative review of theory, empirical support, and call for new directions. *Women's Studies International Forum, 62*, 78–82.

Cook, J. (2000). Sexuality and people with disabilities. *Sexuality and Disability, 18*(3), 195–206.

Cooperrider, D., & Whitney, D. (1999). *A positive revolution in change: Appreciative inquiry*. Taos, NM: Corporation for Positive Change.

Copeland, M. (2007). Mary Ellen Copeland-Wellness Recovery Action Planning, part 1 of 2. Retrieved from https://www.youtube.com/watch?v=JOH5fps4Vpo

Corrigan, P., McCorkle, B., Schell, B., & Kidder, K. (2003). Religion and spirituality in the lives of people with serious mental illness. *Community Mental Health Journal, 39*, 487–499.

Corrigan, P., Thompson, V., Lambert, D., Sangster, Y., Noel, J. G., & Campbell, J. (2003). Perceptions of discrimination among persons with serious mental illness. *Psychiatric Services, 54*(8), 1105–1110.

Corrigan, P. W., & Phelan, S. M. (2004). Social support and recovery in people with serious mental illnesses. *Community Mental Health Journal, 40*, 513–523.

Corrigan, P. W., Salzer, M., Ralph, R. O., Sangster, Y., & Keck, L. (2004). Examining the factor structure of the Recovery Assessment Scale. *Schizophrenia Bulletin, 30*(4), 1035–1041.

Corrigan, P. W., Steiner, L., McCracken, S. G., Blaser, B., & Barr, M. (2001). Strategies for disseminating evidence-based practices to staff who treat people with serious mental illness. *Psychiatric Services, 52*(12), 1598–1606.

Craig, M., & Abel, K. (2001). Drugs in pregnancy: Prescribing for psychiatric disorders in pregnancy and lactation. *Best Practices & Research: Clinical Obstetrics & Gynaecology, 15*, 1013–1030.

Crenshaw, K. (1993). Demarginalizing the intersection of race and sex: A Black feminist critique of antidiscrimination doctrine, feminist theory and antiracist politics. In D. K. Weisberg (Ed.), *Feminist legal theory* (pp. 383–395). Philadelphia, PA: Temple University Press.

Crowther, R. Marshall, M. Bond, G., & Huxley, P. (2001). Vocational rehabilitation for people with severe mental illness. *Cochrane Database Systematic Reviews, 2*, CD003080.

Cunningham, P., McKenzie, K., & Taylor, E. F. (2006). The struggle to provide community-based care to low-income people with serious mental illnesses. *Health Affairs, 25*(3), 694–705.

Cusack, K. J., Grubaugh, A. L., Knapp, R. G., & Frueh, B. C. (2006). Unrecognized trauma and PTSD among public mental health consumers with chronic and severe mental illness. *Community Mental Health Journal, 42*, 487–500.

Cusack, K. J., Morrisey, J. P., & Ellis, A. R. (2008). Targeting trauma-related interventions and improving outcomes for women with co-occurring disorders. *Administration and Policy in Mental Health, 35*(3), 147–158.

Cusack, P., Cusack, F. P., McAndrew, S., McKeown, M., & Duxbury J. (2018). An integrative review exploring the physical and psychological harm inherent in using restraint in mental health inpatient settings. *International Journal of Mental Health Nursing, 27*(3), 1162–1176.

Dakota-Lakota-Nakota Human Rights Advocacy Coalition. (2011). Retrieved from http://www.dlncoalition.org/home.htm

Daniel, W. A. (2003). Mechanisms of cellular distribution of psychotropic drugs: Significance for drug action and interactions. *Progress in Neuro-Psychopharmacology & Biological Psychiatry, 27*, 65–73.

Davidson, L., Haghund, K., Stayner, D., Rakfeldt, J., Chinman, M., & Tebes, J. (2001). "It was just realizing . . . that life isn't one big horror": A qualitative study of supported socialization. *Psychiatric Rehabilitation Journal, 24*, 275–292.

Davidson, L., O'Connell, M. J., Tondora, J., Staeheli, M. R., & Evans, A. C. (2005). Recovery in serious mental illness: A new wine or just a new bottle? *Professional Psychology: Research and Practice, 3*, 480–487.

Davidson, L., & Roe, D. (2007). Recovery from versus recovery in serious mental illness: One strategy for lessening confusion plaguing recovery. *Journal of Mental Health, 16*(4), 459–470.

Davidson, L., Tondora, J., O'Connell, M., Kirk, T., Rockholz, P., & Evans, A. C. (2007). Creating a recovery-oriented system of behavioral health care: Moving from concept to reality. *Psychiatric Rehabilitation Journal, 31*, 23–31.

Davidson, L., & White, W. (2007). The concept of recovery as an organizing principle for integrating mental health and addiction services. *Journal of Behavioral Health Services & Research, 34*(2), 109–120.

Davis, B. (2005). Mediators of the relationship between hope and well-being in older adults. *Clinical Nursing Research, 14,* 253–272.

Davis, M., & Vander Stoep, A. (1997). The transition to adulthood for youth who have serious emotional disturbance: Developmental transition and young adult outcomes. *Journal of Mental Health Administration, 24*(4), 400–427.

Davison, J., & Huntington, A. (2010). "Out of sight": Sexuality and women with enduring mental illness. *International Journal of Mental Health Nursing, 19,* 240–249.

Dawes, M., & Chowienczyk, P. J. (2001). Drugs in pregnancy: Pharmacokinetics in pregnancy. *Best Practices & Research: Clinical Obstetrics & Gynaecology, 15,* 819–826.

Deegan, P. (2011). Spiritual lessons in recovery. Retrieved from http://www/patdeegan.com/blog/archives/000011.php

Deegan, P. E. (2001). *Human sexuality and mental illness: Consumer viewpoints and recovery principles.*

Deegan, P. E., Rapp, C., Holter, M., & Riefer, M. (2008). Best practices: A program to support shared decision making in an outpatient psychiatric medication clinic. *Psychiatric Services, 59*(6), 603–605.

DeGruy, J. (2005). *Posttraumatic slave syndrome: America's legacy of enduring injury and healing.* Portland, OR: Uptone.

DeHert, M., Correll, C. U., Bobes, J., Cetkovich-Bakmas, M., Cohen, D., Asai, I., . . . Leucht, S. (2011). Physical illness in patients with severe mental disorders. I. Prevalence, impact of medications and disparities in health care. *World Psychiatry, 10,* 52–77.

de Jong, S., van Donkersgoed, R. J. M., Timmerman, M. E., Aan Het Rot, M., Wunderink, L., Arends, J., . . . Pijnenborg, G. H. M. (2019). Metacognitive reflection and insight therapy (MERIT) for patients with schizophrenia. *Psychological Medicine, 49*(2), 303–313.

Della-Giustina, K., & Chow, G. (2003). Medications in pregnancy and lactation. *Emergency Medicine Clinics of North America, 21,* 585–613.

Desmond, M. (2016). *Evicted.* Washington, DC: Crown Books.

Diaz-Caneja, A., & Johnson, S. (2004). The views and experiences of severely mentally ill mothers: A qualitative study. *Social Psychiatry and Psychiatric Epidemiology, 39,* 472–482.

Dickerson, F. B., Brown, C. B., Kreyenbuhl, J., Goldberg, R. W., Fang, L. J., & Dixon, L. B. (2004). Sexual and reproductive behaviors among persons with mental illness. *Psychiatric Services, 55,* 1299–1301.

Dixon, L., Adams, C., & Lucksted, A. (2000). Update on family psychoeducation for schizophrenia. *Schizophrenia Bulletin, 26*(1), 5–20.

Dixon, L., McFarlane, W. R., Lefley, H., Lucksted, A., Cohen, M., Falloon, I., . . . Sondheimer, D. (2001). Evidence-based practices for services to families of people with psychiatric disabilities. *Psychiatric Services, 52,* 903–910.

Dixon, L. B., Dickerson, F., Bellack, A. S., Bennett, M., Dickinson, D., Goldberg, R. W., . . . Peer, J. (2009). The 2009 schizophrenia PORT psychosocial treatment recommendations and summary statements. *Schizophrenia Bulletin, 36*(1), 48–70.

Dobson, K. S., & Dozois, D. J. A. (2010). Historical and philosophical bases of the cognitive-behavioral therapies. In K. Dobson (Ed.), *Handbook of cognitive-behavioral therapies* (pp. 3–38). New York, NY: Guilford Press.

Dohrenwend, B. P., Levav, I., Shrout, P. E., Schwartz, S., Naveh, G., Link, B. G., . . . Stueve, A. (1992). Socioeconomic status and psychiatric disorders: The causation-selection issue. *Science, 255*(5047), 946–952.

Doucet, S., Jones, I., Letourneau, N., Dennis, C., & Blackmore, E. R. (2011). Interventions for the prevention and treatment of postpartum psychosis: A systematic review. *Archives of Women's Mental Health, 14,* 89–98.

Drake, R. E., Deegan, P. E., & Rapp, C. (2010). The promise of shared decision making in mental health. *Psychiatric Rehabilitation Journal, 34,* 7–13.

Drew, N., Funk, M., Tang, S., Lamichhane, J., Chávez, E., & Katontoka, S. (2011). Human rights violations of people with mental and psychosocial disabilities: An unresolved global crisis. *Global Mental Health, 378*(9803), 1664–1675.

Duckworth, M. P., & Follette, V. M. (2013). *Retraumatization: Assessment, treatment, and prevention.* New York, NY: Routledge.

Dutton, M. A., Bermudez, D., Matas, A., Majid, H., & Myers, N. L. (2013). Mindfulness-based stress reduction for low-income, predominantly African American women with PTSD and a history of intimate partner violence. *Cognitive and Behavioral Practice, 20*(1), 23–32.

Eack, S. M., & Newhill, C. E., 2007. Psychiatric symptoms and quality of life in schizophrenia: A meta-analysis. *Schizophrenia Bulletin, 33,* 1225–1237.

Elbaz-Haddad, M., & Savaya, R. (2011). Effectiveness of a psychosocial intervention model for persons with chronic psychiatric disorders in long-term hospitalization. *Evaluative Review, 35,* 379–398.

Enns, C. (2004). *Feminist theories and feminist psychotherapies: Origins, themes, and diversity.* New York, NY: Haworth Press.

Eriksen, K., & Kress, V. E. (2008). Gender and diagnosis: Struggles and suggestions for counselors. *Journal of Counseling and Development, 86,* 152–162.

Ernst, C. L., & Goldberg, J. F. (2002). The reproductive safety profile of mood stabilizers, atypical antipsychotics, and broad-spectrum psychotropics. *Journal of Clinical Psychiatry, 63*(4), 42–55.

Fallot, R. D. (2007). Spirituality and religion in recovery: Some current issues. *Psychiatric Rehabilitation Journal, 30*(4), 261–270.

Fallot, R. D. (2008). Spirituality and religion. In K. T. Mueser & D. V. Jeste (Eds.), *Clinical handbook of schizophrenia* (pp. 592–603). New York, NY: Guilford Press.

Farina, A., Allen, J. G., & Saul, B. B. (1968). The role of the stigmatized in affecting social relationships. *Journal of Personality, 36,* 169–182.

Farina, A., Gliha, D., Boudreau, L., Allen, J., & Sherman, M. (1971). Mental illness and the impact of believing others know about it. *Journal of Abnormal Psychology, 77,* 1–5.

Fazel, S., & Danesh, J. (2002). Serious mental disorder in 23,000 prisoners: A systematic review of 62 surveys. *Lancet, 359*(9306), 545–550.

Felker, B., Yazel, J. J., & Short, D. (1996). Mortality and medical comorbidity among psychiatric patients: A review. *Psychiatric Services, 47,* 1356–1363.

Figley, C. R. (1995). *Compassion fatigue: Coping with secondary traumatic stress disorder in those who treat the traumatized.* New York, NY: Brunner-Routledge.

Fischbach, R. L., & Herbert, B. (1997). Domestic violence and mental health: Correlates and conundrums within and across cultures. *Social Science and Medicine, 45,* 1161–1170.

Flaskerud, J. H., & Hu, L. (1992). Relationship of ethnicity to psychiatric diagnosis. *Journal of Nervous and Mental Disease, 180,* 296–303.

Foa, E. B., & Street, G. P. (2001). Women and traumatic events. *Journal of Clinical Psychiatry, 62,* 29–34.

Ford, J. (2007). *Trauma affect regulation: Guide for education and therapy.* University of Connecticut Health Center.

Frech, A., & Damaske, S. (2012). The relationships between mothers' work pathways and physical and mental health. *Journal of Health and Social Behavior, 53*(4), 396–412.

Frederick, D. E., & VanderWeele, T. J. (2019). Supported employment: Meta-analysis and review of randomized controlled trials of individual placement and support. *PLoS One, 14*(2), e0212208.

Fredrickson, B. L., & Roberts, T. (1997). Objectification theory: Toward understanding women's lived experiences and mental health risks. *Psychology of Women Quarterly, 21,* 173–206.

Fredrickson, B. L., Roberts, T., Noll, S. M., Quinn, D. M., & Twenge, J. M. (1998). That swimsuit becomes you: Sex differences in self-objectification, restrained eating, and math performance. *Journal of Personality and Social Psychology, 75,* 269–284.

Frederiksen, M. C. (2001). Physiologic changes in pregnancy and their effect on drug disposition. *Seminars in Perinatology, 25,* 120–123.

Friedman, S., & Harrison, G. (1984). Sexual histories, attitudes and behavior of schizophrenic and normal women. *Archives of Sexual Behavior, 13,* 555–567.

Friedman, S. H., Kaplan, R. S., Rosenthal, M. B., & Console, P. (2010). Music therapy in perinatal psychiatry: Use of lullabies for pregnant and postpartum women with mental illness. *Music and Medicine, 2*(4), 219–225.

Frueh, B. C., Dalton, M. E., Johnson, M. R., Hiers, T. G., Gold, P. B., Magruder, K. M., & Santos, A. B. (2000). Trauma within the psychiatric setting: Conceptual framework, research directions, and policy implications. *Administration and Policy in Mental Health, 28,* 147–154.

Frueh, B. C., Knapp, R. G., Cusack, K. J., Grubaugh, A. L., Sauvageot, J. A., Cousins, V. C., . . . Hiers, T. G. (2005). Special section on seclusion and restraint: Patients' reports of traumatic or harmful experiences within the psychiatric setting. *Psychiatric Services, 56*(9), 1123–1133.

Gabbidon, J., Farrelly, S., Hatch, S. L., Hendeson, C., Williams, P., Bhugra, D., . . . Clement, S. (2014). Discrimination attributed to mental illness or race-ethnicity by users of community psychiatric services. *Psychiatric Services, 65,* 1360–1366.

Gex-Fabry, M., Balant-Gorgia, A. E., & Balant, L. P. (2001). Therapeutic drug monitoring databases for postmarketing surveillance of drug interactions. *Drug Safety, 24,* 947–959.

Gjere, N. A. (2001). Psychopharmacology in pregnancy. *Journal of Perinatal & Neonatal Nursing, 14,* 12–25.

Glynn, S., Marder, S., Cohen, A., Hamilton, A., Saks, E., Hollan, D., & Brekke, J. (2010). *How do some people with schizophrenia thrive?* Paper presentation. American Psychological Association Convention, San Diego, CA.

Goldberg, R. W., Rollins, A. L., & Lehman, A. F. (2003). Social network correlates among people with psychiatric disabilities. *Psychiatric Rehabilitation Journal, 26*(4), 393–402.

Goodell, W. (1882). Extirpation of the ovaries for insanity. *Medical and Surgical Reporter, 46*(21), 575.

Goodman, L. A., Dutton, M. A., & Harris, M. (1995). Episodically homeless women with serious mental illness: Prevalence of physical and sexual assault. *American Journal of Orthopsychiatry, 65*, 468–478.

Goodman, L. A., Salyers, M. P., Mueser, K. T., Rosenberg, S. D., Swartz, M., Essock, S., . . . Swanson, J. (2001). Recent victimization in women and men with severe mental illness: Prevalence and correlates. *Journal of Traumatic Stress, 14*, 615–632.

Goodman, L., Thompson, K., Weinfurt, K., Corl, S., Acker, P., Mueser, K., & Rosenberg, S. D. (1999). Reliability of reports of violent victimization and posttraumatic stress disorder among men and women with serious mental illness. *Journal of Traumatic Stress, 12*, 587–599.

Gove, W. R. (1980). Mental illness and psychiatric treatment among women. *Psychology of Women Quarterly, 4*(3), 345–362.

Gove, W. R. (1984). Gender differences in mental and physical illness: The effects of fixed roles and nurturant roles. *Social Science & Medicine, 19*(2), 77–84.

Graff, L. A., Dyck, D. G., & Schallow, J. R. (1991). Predicting postpartum depressive symptoms: A structural modeling analysis. *Perceptual and Motor Skills, 73*, 1137–1138.

Greenberg, J. S., Greenley, J. R., & Benedict, P. (1994). Contributions of persons with serious mental illness to their families. *Psychiatric Services, 45*(5), 475–480.

Gressier, F., Guillard, V., Cazas, O., Falissard, B., Glangeaud-Freudenthal, N. M., & Sutter-Dallay, A. L. (2017). Risk factors for suicide attempt in pregnancy and the post-partum period in women with serious mental illnesses. *Journal of Psychiatric Research, 84*, 284–291.

Groneman, C. (1994). The historical construction of female sexuality. *Signs, 19*(2), 337–367.

Groneman, C. (2001). *Nymphomania: A history.* New York, NY: Norton.

Gudjonsson, G. H., Savona, C. S. V., Green, T., & Terry, R. (2011). The recovery approach to the care of mentally disordered patients: Does it predict treatment engagement and positive social behaviour beyond quality of life? *Personality and Individual Differences, 51*, 899–903.

Gupta, U., & Gupta, B. S. (2014). Religious involvement, well-being, and mental health in men and women. *Journal of Psychosocial Research, 9*(1), 179–202.

Hanna, F. J., & Green, A. (2004). Asian shades of spirituality: Toward an integrated approach to psychotherapy. *Professional School Counseling, 7*, 326–333.

Hardy, K., & Laszloffy, T. A. (1995). The cultural genogram: Key to training culturally competent family therapists. *Journal of Marital and Family Therapy, 21*(3), 227–237.

Harris, R. Z., Benet, L. Z., & Schwartz, J. B. (1995). Gender effects in pharmacokinetics and pharmacodynamics. *Drugs, 50*, 222–239.

Harris, M., & Landis, C. (Eds.). *Sexual abuse in the lives of women with serious mental illness.* New York, NY: Brunner-Routledge.

Harrison, G., Croudace, T., Mason, P., Glazebrook, C., & Medley, I. (1996). Predicting the long-term outcome of schizophrenia. *Psychological Medicine, 26*, 697–705.

Hatton, E., & Trautner, M. N. (2011). Equal opportunity objectification? The sexualization of men and women on the cover of Rolling Stone. *Sexuality & Culture, 15*(3), 256–278.

Heath, C. D. (2006). A womanist approach to understanding and assessing the relationship between spirituality and mental health. *Mental Health, Religion & Culture, 9*(2), 155–170.

Hellman, R. E., & Klein, E. (2004). A program for lesbian, gay, bisexual, and transgender individuals with major mental illness. *Journal of Gay & Lesbian Psychotherapy, 8*(3–4), 67–82.

Hellman, R. E., Klein, E., Huygen, C., Chew, M., & Uttaro, T. (2010). A program for lesbian, gay, bisexual, and transgender individuals with major mental illness, *Best Practices in Mental Health, 6*(12), 13–26.

Hellman, R. E., Sudderth, L., & Avery, A. M. (2002). Major mental illness in a sexual minority psychiatric sample. *Journal of the Gay and Lesbian Medical Association, 6*(3/4), 97–106.

Hendryx, M., Green, C. A., & Perrin, N. A. (2009). Social support, activities, and recovery from serious mental illness: STARS study findings. *Journal of Behavioral Health Services & Research, 36*(3), 320–329.

Herman, J. (1997). *Trauma and recovery.* New York, NY: Perseus Books Group.

Hirshbein, L. (2006). Science, gender, and the emergence of depression in American Psychiatry, 1952–1980. *Journal of the History of Medicine and Allied Sciences, 61*(2), 187–216.

Hirshbein, L. (2010). Sex and gender in psychiatry: A view from history. *Journal of Medical Humanities, 32*(2), 155–170.

Hobfoll, S., Ritter, C., Lavin, J., Hulsizer, M. R., & Cameron, R. P. (1995). Depression prevalence and incidence among inner-city pregnant and postpartum women. *Journal of Consulting Clinical Psychology, 63*, 445–53.

Hochschild, A., & Machung, A. (2003). *The second shift: Working parents and the revolution at home.* New York, NY: Penguin Group Inc.

Hogan, R. (1980). *Human sexuality: A nursing perspective.* New York, NY: Appleton-Century-Crofts.

Homel, P., Casey, D., & Allison, D. B. (2002). Changes in body mass index for individuals with and without schizophrenia. *Schizophrenia Research, 55*, 277–284.

Horwitz, A. V., Reinhard, S. C., & Howell-White, S. (1996). Caregiving as reciprocal exchange in families with seriously mentally ill members. *Journal of Health and Social Behavior, 37*(2), 149–162.

Hudson, C. G. (2005). Socioeconomic status and mental illness: Tests of the social causation and selection hypotheses. *American Journal of Orthopsychiatry, 75*(1), 3–18.

Ida, D. J. (2007). Cultural competency and recovery within diverse populations. *Psychiatric Rehabilitation Journal, 31*(1), 49–53.

Jablensky, A., Sartorius, N., Ernberg, G., Anker, M., Korten, A., Cooper, J. E., . . . Bertelsen, A. (1992). Schizophrenia: Manifestations, incidence and course in different cultures. A World Health Organization Ten-Country Study. *Psychological Medicine Monograph Supplement, 20*, 1–97.

Jennings, A. (2009). Retraumatization. Retrieved from www.theannainstitute.org

Johnson, S., Lamb, D., Marston, L., Osborn, D., Mason, O., Henderson, C., . . . Sullivan, S. (2018). Peer-supported self-management for people discharged from a mental health crisis team: A randomised controlled trial. *Lancet, 392*(10145), 409–418.

Jonikas, J. A., Grey, D. D., Copeland, M. E., Razzano, L. A., Hamilton, M. M., Floyd, C. B., . . . Cook, J. A. (2013). Improving propensity for patient self-advocacy through wellness recovery action planning: results of a randomized controlled trial. *Community Mental Health Journal, 49*(3), 260–269.

Jonikas, J. A., Laris, A., & Cook, J. A. (2003). The passage to adulthood: Psychiatric rehabilitation service and transition-related needs of young adult women with emotional and psychiatric disorders. *Psychiatric Rehabilitation Journal, 27*(2), 114–121.

Kaschak, E. (1992). *Engendered lives: A new psychology of women's experience.* New York, NY: Basic Books.

Kashuba, A. D., & Nafziger, A. N. (1998). Physiological changes during the menstrual cycle and their effects on the pharmacokinetics and pharmacodynamics of drugs. *Clinical Pharmacokinetics, 34,* 203–218.

Kendler, K. S., Walters, E. E., & Kessler, R. C. (1997). The prediction of length of major depressive episodes: Results from an epidemiological sample of female twins. *Psychological Medicine, 27,* 107–117.

Kessler, R. C., & Üstün, T. B. (Eds.) (2008). *The WHO world mental health surveys: Global perspectives on the epidemiology of mental disorders.* New York, NY: Cambridge University Press.

Khandelwal, S. K., Jhingan, H. P., Ramesh, S., Gupta, R. K., & Srivastava, V. K. (2004). India mental health country profile. *International Review of Psychiatry, 16*(1–2), 126–141.

Khantzian, E. J. (2012). Reflections on treating addictive disorders: A psychodynamic perspective. *American Journal on Addictions, 21,* 274–279.

Kidd, S. A., McKenzie, K., Collins, A., Clark, C., Costa, L, Mihalakakos, B. A., & Paterson, J. (2014). Advancing the recovery orientation of hospital care through staff engagement with former clients of inpatient units. *Psychiatric Services, 65*(2), 221–225.

Kidd, S. A., McKenzie, K. J., & Virdee, G. (2014). Mental health reform at a systems level: Widening the lens on recovery-oriented care. *Canadian Journal of Psychiatry, 59*(5), 243–249.

Kidd, S. A., Veltman, A., Gately, C., Chan, K. J., & Cohen, J. N. (2011). Lesbian, gay, and transgender persons with severe mental illness: Negotiating wellness in the context of multiple sources of stigma. *American Journal of Psychiatric Rehabilitation, 14*(1), 13–39.

Kidd, S. A., Virdee, G., Kurpa, T., Burnham, D., Hemingway, D., Margolin, I., . . . Zabkiewicz, D. (2013). The role of gender in housing for individuals with severe mental illness: A qualitative study of the Canadian service context. *British Medical Journal Open, 3*(6), e002914.

Kilpatrick, D., Resnick, H. S., Milanak, M. E., Miller, M. W., Keys, K. M., & Friedman, M. J. (2013). National estimates of exposure to potentially traumatic events and PTSD prevalence using DSM-IV and DSM-5 criteria. *Journal of Traumatic Stress, 26,* 537–547.

Kirsh, B. (2000). Factors associated with employment for mental health consumers. *Psychiatric Rehabilitation Journal, 24*(1), 13–21.

Kirst, M., Zerger, S., Harris, D. W., Plenert, E., & Stergiopoulos, V. (2014). The promise of recovery: Narratives of hope among homeless individuals with mental illness participating in a Housing First randomized controlled trial in Toronto, Canada. *British Medical Journal, 4,* e004379.

Kleiber, B. V., Felder, J. F., Ashby, B., Scott, S., Dean, J., & Dimidjian, S. (2017). Treating depression among adolescent perinatal women with a dialectical behavior therapy-informed skills group. *Cognitive and Behavioral Practice, 24*, 416–427.

Kleinman, A. (1988). *The illness narratives: Suffering, healing, and the human condition.* New York, NY: Basic Books.

Klontz, B., Britt, S. L., Mentzer, J., & Klontz, T. (2011). Money beliefs and financial behaviors: Development of the Klontz Money Script Inventory. *Journal of Financial Therapy, 2*(1), 1–22.

Ko, S., J., Ford, J. D., Kassam-Adams, N., Berkowitz, S. J., Wilson, C., Wong, M., ... Layne, C. M. (2008). Creating trauma-informed systems: Child welfare, education, first responders, health care, Juvenile justice. *Professional Psychology: Research & Practice, 39*, 396–404.

Koenig, H. G. (1998). *Handbook of religion and mental health.* New York, NY: Oxford University Press.

Kohn-Wood, L. P., & Wilson, M. N. (2005). The context of caretaking in rural areas: Family factors influencing the level of functioning of seriously mentally ill Patients living at home. *American Journal of Community Psychology, 36*(1/2), 1–13.

Kramer, M. (1954). The 1951 survey of the use of psychosurgery. In W. Overholser (Ed.), *Proceedings of the Third Research Conference on Psychosurgery, Public Health Service Publication* (pp. 159–168). Washington, DC: U.S. Government Printing Office.

Kreyenbuhl, J., Buchanan, R. W., Dickerson, F. B., & Dixon, L. B. (2010). The schizophrenia patient outcomes research team (PORT): Updated treatment recommendations 2009. *Schizophrenia Bulletin, 36*, 94–103.

Kuruvilla, A., Peedicayil, J., Srikrishna, G., Kuruvilla, K., & Kanagasabapathy, A. S. (1992). A study of serum prolactin levels in schizophrenia: Comparison of males and females. *Clinical and Experimental Pharmacology and Physiology, 19*, 603–606.

LaFramboise, T. D., Trimble, J. E., & Monatt, G. V. (1990). Counseling intervention and American Indian tradition: An integrative approach. *Counseling Psychologist, 18*, 628–654.

Landeen, J., Pawlick, J., Woodside, H., Kirkpatrick, H., & Byrne, C. (2000). Hope, quality of life, and symptom severity in individuals with schizophrenia. *Psychiatric Rehabilitation Journal, 23*, 364–369.

Larkin, W., & Morrison, A. P. (2006). Relationships between trauma and psychosis: From theory to therapy. In W. Larkin & A. P. Morrison (Eds.), *Trauma and psychosis: New directions for theory and therapy* (pp. 259–282). New York, NY: Routledge.

Lauver, D. R. (2000). Commonalities in women's spirituality and women's health. *Advances in Nursing Science, 22*(3), 76–88.

Lecomte, T. (2018). Group cognitive behavioural therapy for people experiencing psychosis. In *Group Therapy for Psychoses* (pp. 137–145).

Lefley, H. P. (2009). *Family psychoeducation for serious mental illness.* New York, NY: Oxford University Press.

Leibowitz, S., & Telingator, C. (2012). Assessing gender identity concerns in children and adolescents: Evaluation, treatments, and outcomes. *Current Psychiatry Reports, 14*, 111–120.

Lennon, M. C., & Rosenfield, S. (1992). Women and mental health: The interaction of job and family conditions. *Journal of Health and Social Behavior, 33*(4), 316–327.

Levin, B. L., & Becker, M. A. (2010). *A public health perspective of women's mental health.* New York, NY: Springer.

Lewis-Hall, F., Williams, T. S., Panetta, J. A., & Herrera, J. M. (Eds.). (2002). *Psychiatric illness in women: Emerging treatments and research.* Washington, DC: American Psychiatric Press.

Linehan, M. M. (2014). *DBT skills training handouts and worksheets.* New York, NY: Guilford Publications.

Link, B. G. (1987). Understanding labeling effects in the area of mental disorders: An assessment of the effects of expectations of rejection. *American Sociological Review, 52,* 96–112.

Lipschitz, D. S., Kaplan, M. L., Sorkenn, J. B., Faeda, G. L., Chorney, P., & Asnis, G. M. (1996). Prevalence and characteristics of physical and sexual abuse among psychiatric outpatients. *Psychiatric Services, 47,* 189–191.

Lloyd, S., & Mizock, L. (2018, August). *Qualitative analysis of strengths among women with serious mental illness.* Poster presented at American Psychological Association Convention, San Francisco, CA.

Lo, C. C., & Cheng, T. C. (2014). Race, unemployment rate, and chronic mental illness: A 15-year trend analysis. *Social Psychiatry and Psychiatric Epidemiology, 49,* 1119–1128.

Lo, C. C., Cheng, T. C., & Howell, R. J. (2014). Access to and utilization of health services as pathway to racial disparities in serious mental illness. *Community Mental Health Journal, 50,* 251–257.

Logie, C. H., James, L., Tharao W., & Loutfy, M. R. (2011). HIV, gender, race, sexual orientation, and sex work: A qualitative study of intersectional stigma experienced by HIV-positive women in Ontario, Canada. *PLoS Medicine, 8*(11), 1–12.

Logsdon, M. C., Wisner, K., Billings, D. M., & Shanahan, B. (2006). Raising the awareness of primary care providers about postpartum depression. *Issues in Mental Health Nursing, 27,* 59–73.

Loughnan, S., Pina, A., Vasquez, E. A., & Puvia, E. (2013). Sexual objectification increases rape victim blame and decreases perceived suffering. *Psychology of Women Quarterly, 37*(4), 455–461.

Lucksted, A. (2004). Lesbian, gay, bisexual, and transgender people receiving services in the public mental health system: Raising issues. *Journal of Gay & Lesbian Psychotherapy, 8*(3/4), 25–42.

Lukoff, D. (2007). Spirituality in the recovery from persistent mental disorders. *Southern Medical Association, 100*(6), 642–646.

MacDonald, E., Sauer, K., Howie, L., & Albiston, D. (2005). What happens to social relationships in early psychosis? *Journal of Mental Health, 14*(2), 129–143.

Malcolm, W., DeCourville, N., & Belicki, K. (2008). *Women's reflections on the complexities of forgiveness.* New York, NY: Routledge.

Mancini, M. A. (2007). The role of self-efficacy in recovery from serious psychiatric disabilities: A qualitative study with fifteen psychiatric survivors. *Qualitative Social Work, 6*(1), 49–74.

Manuel, J. I., Hinterland, K., Conover, S., & Herman, D. B. (2012). "I hope I can make it out there": Perceptions of women with severe mental illness on the transition from hospital to community. *Community Mental Health Journal, 48*(3), 302–308.

Marzolini, S., Jensen, B., & Melville, P. (2009). Feasibility and effects of a group-based re-
    sistance and aerobic exercise program for individuals with severe schizophrenia: A
    multidisciplinary approach. *Mental Health and Physical Activity*, 2, 29–36.

Mauritz, M. W., Goossens, P. J., Draijer, N., & van Achterberg, T. (2013). Prevalence of
    interpersonal trauma exposure and trauma-related disorders in severe mental ill-
    ness. *European Journal of Psychotraumatology*, 4. doi:10.3402/ejpt.v4i0.19985

Mays, V. M., & Cochran, S. D. (2001). Mental health correlates of perceived discrimina-
    tion among lesbian, gay, and bisexual adults in the United States. *American Journal
    of Public Health*, 91(11), 1869–1876.

McCall, L. (2005). The complexity of intersectionality. *Journal of Women and Culture in
    Society*, 30(3), 1771–1800.

McCann, I. L., & Pearlman, L. A. (1990). Vicarious traumatization: A framework for un-
    derstanding the psychological effects of working with victims. *Journal of Traumatic
    Stress*, 3(1), 131–149.

McCorkle, B. H., Rogers, E. S., Dunn, E. C., Lyass, A., & Wan, Y. M. (2008). Increasing
    social support for individuals with serious mental illness: Evaluating the compeer
    model of intentional friendship. *Community Mental Health Journal*, 44(5), 359–366.

McCreadie, R. G. (1982). The Nithsdale schizophrenia survey: I. Psychiatric and social
    handicaps. *British Journal of Psychiatry*, 140, 582–586.

McFarlane, A. C., Bookless, C., & Air, T. (2001). Posttraumatic stress disorder in a ge-
    neral psychiatric inpatient population. *Journal of Traumatic Stress*, 14, 633–645.

McGovern, C. M. (1981). Doctors or ladies? Women physicians in psychiatric
    institutions, 1872–1900. *Bulletin of the History of Medicine*, 55(10), 88–107.

McGovern, P., Dowd, B., Gjerdingen, D., Gross, C. R., Kenney, S., Ukestad,
    L., . . . Lundberg, U. (2006). Postpartum health of employed mothers 5 weeks after
    childbirth. *Annals of Family Medicine*, 4, 159–167.

Meade, C. S., & Sikkema, K. J. (2005). HIV risk behavior among adults with severe
    mental illness: A systematic review. *Clinical Psychology Review*, 25, 433–457.

Meltzer, H. Y., Rabinowitz, J., Lee, M. A., Cola, P. A., Ranjan, R., Findling, R. L., &
    Thompson, P. A. (1997). Age at onset and gender of schizophrenic patients in rela-
    tion to neuroleptic resistance. *American Journal of Psychiatry*, 154, 475–482.

Mercer, J. (2012). Child myths blog: A spin-off of Mercer's book, "Thinking critically
    about child development: Examining myths & misunderstandings." Retrieved from
    http://childmyths.blogspot.com/2012/01/shades-of-snake-pit-wet-pack-is-back.
    html

Meyer, I. (2003). Prejudice, social stress and mental health in lesbian, gay, and bisexual
    populations: Conceptual issues and research evidence. *Psychological Bulletin*, 129,
    674–697.

Mezzina, R., Davidson, L., Borg, M., Marin, I., Topor, A., & Sells, D. (2006). The social
    nature of recovery. *American Journal of Psychiatric Rehabilitation*, 9, 63–80.

Michélsen, H., 2002. Gender differences in the effects from working: Conditions in
    mental health: A 4-year follow-up. *International Archives of Occupational and
    Environmental Health*, 75, 252–258.

Miech, R. A., Caspi, A. Moffitt, T. E., Entner Wright, B. R., & Silva, P. A. (1999). Low so-
    cioeconomic status and mental disorders: A longitudinal study of selection and cau-
    sation during young adulthood. *American Journal of Sociology*, 104(4), 1096–113.

Miller, J., & Stiver, I. (1997). *The healing connection: How women form relationships in therapy and in life*. Boston, MA: Beacon Press.

Miller, J. B. (2008). VI. Connections, disconnections, and violations. *Feminism & Psychology, 18*(3), 368–380.

Miller, L., & Finnerty, M. (1996). Sexuality, pregnancy, and childrearing among women with schizophrenia-spectrum disorders. *Psychiatric Services, 47*, 502–506.

Miller, M. A. (2001). Gender-based differences in the toxicity of pharmaceuticals—the Food and Drug Administration's perspective. *International Journal of Toxicology, 20*, 149–152.

Miller, R., & McCormack, J. (2006). Faith and religious delusions in first-episode schizophrenia. *Social Work in Mental Health, 4*(4), 37–50.

Milner, A., King, T., LaMontagne, A., Bentley, R., & Kavanagh, A. (2018). Men's work, women's work, and mental health: A longitudinal investigation of the relationship between the gender composition of occupations and mental health. *Social Science & Medicine, 204*, 16–22.

Mizock, L. (2019). Development of a gender-sensitive and recovery-oriented intervention for women with serious mental illness. *Psychiatric Rehabilitation Journal, 42*(1), 3–8.

Mizock, L., Aitken, D., & LaMar, K. (2019). Work assets and drains: Employment experiences of women with serious mental illness. *Journal of Vocational Rehabilitation, 50*, 193–205.

Mizock, L., & Brubaker, M. (In press). *Diagnostic re-ordering: Mental health treatment experiences of women with serious mental illness*. Psychological Services.

Mizock, L., DeMartini, L., LaMar, K., & Stringer, J. (2019). Relational resilience: Intimate and romantic relationship experiences of women with serious mental illness. *Journal of Relationships Research, 10*(e5), 1–9.

Mizock, L., & Fleming, M. (2011). Transgender and gender variant populations with mental illness: Implications for clinical care. *Professional Psychology, 42*(2), 208–213.

Mizock, L., & Harkins, D. (2012). *Researcher race: Social constructions in the research process*. Charlotte, NC: Information Age Publishing.

Mizock, L., & Kaschak, E. (2015). Introduction to the special issue: Women with serious mental illness in therapy: Intersectional perspectives. *Women & Therapy, 38*(1-2), 6–13.

Mizock, L., & Lewis, T. K. (2008). Trauma in transgender populations: Risk, resilience, and clinical care. *Journal of Emotional Abuse, 8*(3), 335–354.

Mizock, L., Merg, A. L., Boyle, E. J., & Kompaniez-Dunigan, E. (2019). Motherhood reimagined: Identity status of women with SMI surrounding parenting. *Psychiatric Rehabilitation Journal, 42*(2), 105–112.

M'Mordie, W. K. (1887). *Removal of both ovaries for masturbation and insanity*. Obstetrical Section, February, 208–209.

Mohr, S., & Huguelet, P. (2004). The relationship between schizophrenia and religion and its implications for care. *Swiss Medical Weekly, 134*, 369–376.

Mohr, T. (2015). *Playing big: Find your voice, your mission, your message*. New York, NY: Avery.

Montgomery, P., Tompkins, C., Forchuk, C., & French, S. (2006). Keeping close: Mothering with serious mental illness. *Journal of Advanced Nursing, 54*(1), 20–28.

Moradi, B., & Huang, Y. P. (2008). Objectification theory and psychology of women: A decade of advances and future directions. *Psychology of Women Quarterly, 32*(4), 377–398.

Morgan, C., Burns, T., Fitzpatrick, R., Pinfold, V., & Priebe, S. (2007). Social exclusion and mental health. *British Journal of Psychiatry, 191*, 477–483.

Morrow, M. (2002). Violence and trauma in the lives of women with serious mental illness: Current practices in service provision in British Columbia. British Columbia Centre of Excellence for Women's Health. Vancouver, BC: Canada. Retrieved from http://bccewh.bc.ca/wp-content/uploads/2012/05/2002_Violence-and-Trauma-in-the-Lives-of-Women-with-Mental-Illness.pdf

Moses-Kolko, E. L., & Roth, E. K. (2004). Antepartum and postpartum depression: Healthy mom, healthy baby. *Journal of the American Medical Women's Association, 59*, 181–91.

Mowbray, C. T. (2003). Women and psychiatric rehabilitation practice. *Psychiatric Rehabilitation Journal, 27*(2), 101–103.

Mowbray, C. T., Bybee, D., Harris, S. H., & McCrohan, N. (1995). Predictors of work status and future work orientation in people with psychiatric disability. *Psychiatric Rehabilitation Journal, 19*(2), 17–28.

Mowbray, C. T., Nicholson, J., & Bellamy, C. D. (2003). Psychosocial rehabilitation service needs of women. *Psychiatric Rehabilitation Journal, 27*(2), 104–113.

Mowbray, C. T., Oyserman, D., Bybee, D., MacFarlane, P., & Rueda-Riedle, A. (2001). Life circumstances of mothers with serious mental illnesses. *Psychiatric Rehabilitation Journal, 25*(2), 114.

Mowbray, C. T., Oyserman, D., & Ross, S. (1995). Parenting and the significance of children for women with a serious mental illness. *Journal of Mental Health Administration, 22*(2), 189–200.

Mowbray, C. T., Oyserman, D., Zemencuk, J. K., & Ross, S. R. (1995). Motherhood for women with serious mental illness: Pregnancy, childbirth, and the postpartum period. *American Journal of Orthopsychiatry, 65*(1), 21–38.

Mueser, K. T., & Glynn, S. M. (1995). *Behavioral family therapy for psychiatric disorders.* Boston, MA: Allyn & Bacon.

Mueser, K. T., Goodman, L. A., Trumbetta, S. L., Rosenberg, S. D., Osher, F. C., Vidaver, R., . . . Foy, D. W. (1998). Trauma and posttraumatic stress disorder in severe mental illness. *Journal of Consulting and Clinical Psychology, 66*, 493–499.

Mueser, K. T., Gottlieb, J. D., Xie, H., Lu, W., Yanos, P. T., Rosenberg, S. D., . . . McHugo, G. J. (2015). Evaluation of cognitive restructuring for post-traumatic stress disorder in people with severe mental illness. *British Journal of Psychiatry, 206*(6), 501–508.

Mueser, K. T., McGurk, S. R., Xie, H., Bolton, E. E., Jankowski, M. K., Lu, W., . . . Wolfe, R. (2018). Neuropsychological predictors of response to cognitive behavioral therapy for posttraumatic stress disorder in persons with severe mental illness. *Psychiatry Research, 259*, 110–116.

Mueser, K. T., & Rosenberg, S. D. (2003). Treating the trauma of first-episode psychosis: A PTSD perspective. *Journal of Mental Health, 13*, 103–108.

Mueser, K. T., Rosenberg, S. D., Goodman, L. A., & Trumbetta, S. L. (2002). Trauma, PTSD, and the course of severe mental illness: An interactive model. *Schizophrenia Research, 53*, 123–143.

Mueser, K. T., Salyers, M. P., Rosenberg, S. D., & Butterfield, M. I. (2004). Interpersonal trauma and posttraumatic stress disorder in patients with severe mental illness: Demographic, clinical, and health correlates. *Schizophrenia Bulletin, 30*(1), 45.

Mueser, K. T., & Taylor, K. L. (1997). A cognitive-behavioral approach. In M. Harris & C. Harris (Eds.), *Sexual abuse in the lives of women with serious mental illness* (pp. 67–90). New York, NY: Brunner-Routledge.

Muntaner, C., Eaton, W., Miech, R., & O'Campo, P. (2004). Socioeconomic position and major mental disorders. *Epidemiologic Reviews, 26,* 53–56.

Murray, J. B. (1992). Kleptomania: A review of the research. *Journal of Psychology, 126*(2), 131–138.

Mustanski, B. S., Garofalo, R., & Emerson, E. M. (2010). Mental health disorders, psychological distress, and suicidality in a divers sample of lesbian, gay, bisexual, and transgender youths. *American Journal of Public Health, 100*(12), 2426–2432.

Naidoo, U., Kinon, B. J., Gilmore, J. A., Liu, H., & Halbreich, U. M. (2003). Hyperprolactinemia in response to antipsychotic drugs: Characterization across comparative clinical trials. *Psychoneuroendocrinology, 28*(Suppl 2), 69–82.

National Alliance on Mental Illness. (2019). NAMI family-to-family. Retrieved from https://www.nami.org/Find-Support/NAMI-Programs/NAMI-Family-to-Family

National Institute of Mental Health. (2015). Serious mental illness (SMI) among U.S. adults. Retrieved from https://www.nimh.nih.gov/health/statistics/prevalence/serious-mental-illness-smi-among-us-adults.shtml

National Research Council and Institute of Medicine. (2009). *Depression in parents, parenting, and children.* Washington, DC: National Academies Press.

New Freedom Commission on Mental Health (2003). *Achieving the promise: Transforming mental health care in America. Final Report.* DHHS Pub. No. SMA-03-3832. Rockville, MD.

Nicholson, J., Nason, M., Calabresi, A., & Yando, R. (1999). Fathers with severe mental illness. *American Journal of Orthopsychiatry, 69,* 134–141.

Nickerson, K. J., Helms, J. E., & Terrell, F. (1994). Cultural mistrust, opinions about mental illness, and Black students' attitudes toward seeking psychological help from White counselors. *Journal of Counseling Psychology, 41,* 378–385.

Nishith, P., Mueser, K. T., & Morse, G. A. (2015). A brief intervention for posttraumatic stress disorder in persons with a serious mental illness. *Psychiatric Rehabilitation Journal, 38*(4), 314.

Nuttbrock, L., Hwahng, S., Bockting, W., Rosenblum, A., Mason, M., Macri, M., & Becker, J. (2010). Psychiatric impact of gender-related abuse across the life course of male-to-female transgender persons. *Journal of Sex Research, 47*(1), 12–23.

O'Hare, T., Shen, C., & Sherrer, M. V. (2017). Race, trauma, and suicide attempts: Comparing African American, White, and Hispanic people with severe mental illness. *Best Practices in Mental Health, 12*(2), 96–108.

O'Hare, T., Sherrer, M. V., & Shen, C. (2006). Subjective distress from stressful events and high-risk behaviors as predictors of PTSD symptoms severity in clients with severe mental illness. *Journal of Traumatic Stress, 19,* 375–386.

Okazaki, S. (2000). Treatment delay among Asian-American patients with severe mental illness. *American Journal of Orthopsychiatry, 70*(1), 58–64.

Olson, D., Cioffi, A., Yovanoff, P., & Mank, D. (2000). Gender differences in supported employment. *Mental Retardation, 38*(2), 89–96.

Omachi, Y., & Sumiyoshi, T. (2018). Dose reduction/discontinuation of antipsychotic drugs in psychosis; effect on cognition and functional outcomes. *Frontiers in Psychiatry, 9,* 447.

Ou, Y., Zhou, Y., & Xian, P. (2018). Effect of obstetric fine nursing on pain during natural childbirth and postpartum recovery. *Iranian Journal of Public Health, 47*(11), 1703.

Oyserman, D., Bybee, D., Mowbray, C. T., & Khang, S. (2000). *The meaning of motherhood for women with mental illness.* Unpublished manuscript, University of Michigan, Ann Arbor.

Oyserman, D., Mowbray, C. T., Meares, P. A., & Firminger, K. B. (2000). Parenting among mothers with a serious mental illness. *American Journal of Orthopsychiatry, 70*(3), 296–315.

Padgett, D. K., Henwood, B., Abrams, C., & Drake, R. E. (2008). Social relationships among persons who have experienced serious mental illness, substance abuse, and homelessness: Implications for recovery. *American Journal of Orthopsychiatry, 78*(3), 333–339.

Park, J. M., Solomon, P., & Mandell, D. S. (2006). Involvement in the child welfare system among mothers with serious mental illness. *Psychiatric Services, 57*(4), 493–497.

Patel, V., Araya, de Lima, R., Ludemir, M., & Todd, A. (1999). Women, poverty and common mental disorders in four restructuring societies. *Social Science & Medicine, 49,* 1461–1471.

Patton, S. W., Misri, S., Corral, M. R., Perry, K. F., & Kuan, A. J. (2002). Antipsychotic medication during pregnancy and lactation in women with schizophrenia: Evaluating the risk. *Canadian Journal of Psychiatry, 47,* 959–965.

Perese, E. (1997). Unmet needs of persons with chronic mental illnesses: Relationship to their adaptation to community living. *Issues in Mental Health Nursing, 18*(1), 18–34.

Perese, E. F. (2007). Stigma, poverty, and victimization: Roadblocks to recovery for individuals with severe mental illness. *Journal of the American Psychiatric Nurses Association, 13,* 285–295.

Perkins, R. (1992). Catherine is having a baby. *Feminism and Psychology, 2,* 110–112.

Perrone, K. M., Wright, S. L., & Jackson, Z. V. (2009). Traditional and nontraditional gender roles and work—family interface for men and women. *Journal of Career Development, 36*(1), 8–24.

Peterson, C., & Seligman, M. *Character strengths and virtues.* New York, NY: Oxford University Press.

Pettus-Davis, C., & Epperson, M. W. (2015). From mass incarceration to smart decarceration. Center for Social Development. Retrieved from https://openscholarship.wustl.edu/cgi/viewcontent.cgi?article=1575&context=csd_research

Pevalin, D. J., & Goldberg, D. P. (2003). Social precursors to onset and recovery from episodes of common mental illness. *Psychological Medicine, 33,* 299–306.

Phelan, J., & Link, B. G. (2004). Fear of people with mental illness: The role of personal and impersonal contact and exposure to threat or harm. *Journal of Health and Social Behavior, 45,* 68–80.

Phelan, J. C., Link, B. G., Stueve, A., & Pescosolido, B. (2000). Public conceptions of mental illness in 1950 and 1996: What is mental illness and is it to be feared? *Journal of Health and Social Behavior, 41,* 188–207.

Phillips-Salimi, C. R., Haase, J. E., Kintner, E. K., Monahan, P. O., & Azzouz, F. (2007). Psychometric properties of the Herth Hope Index in adolescents and young adults with cancer. *Journal of Nursing Measures, 15,* 3–23.

Pinderhughes, C. A., Barrabee, E., & Reyna, L. J. (1972). Psychiatric disorders and sexual functioning. *American Journal of Psychiatry*, *128*, 1276–1283.

Ponce, A. N., & Rowe, M. (2018). Citizenship and community mental health care. *American Journal of Community Psychology*, *61*(1-2), 22–31.

Porter, R. (2002). *Madness: A brief history*. New York, NY: Oxford University Press.

Prichard, I., & Tiggemann, M. (2005). Objectification in fitness centers: Self- objectification, body dissatisfaction, and disordered eating in aerobic instructors and aerobic participants. *Sex Roles*, *53*, 19–28.

Primm, A. B., Vasquez, M. J. T., Mays, R. A., Sammons-Posey, D., McKnight-Eily, L. R., Presley-Cantrell, L. R., . . . Perry, G. S. (2010). The role of public health in addressing racial and ethnic disparities in mental health and mental illness. *Preventing Chronic Disease*, *7*(1), A20.

Probate Courts of Connecticut. (2008). Guidelines for conservators. Retrieved from https://www.laws.com/uploads/cms/20101110/4cdaecafccdeb.pdf

Rapetti, M., Carta, M. G., & Fadda, B. (2012). *Clinical Practice & Epidemiology in Mental Health*, *8*, 110–119.

Read, J., Agar, K., Argyle, N., & Aderhold, V. (2003). Sexual and physical abuse during childhood and adulthood as predictors of hallucinations, delusions and thought disorder. *Psychology and Psychotherapy: Theory, Research and Practice*, *76*(1), 1–22.

Reilly, M. A. (1997). A question of illness, injustice, or both? In M. Harris & C. Landis (Eds.), *Sexual abuse in the lives of women diagnosed with serious mental illness*. New York, NY: Brunner-Routledge.

Repetti, R. L., Matthews, K. A., & Waldron, I. (1989). Effects of paid employment on women's mental and physical health. *American Psychologist*, *44*(11), 1394–1401.

Resick, P. A., Bovin, M. J., Calloway, A. L., Dick, A. M., King, M. W., Mitchell, K. S., . . . Wolf, E. J. (2013). A critical evaluation of the complex PTSD literature: Implications for DSM-5. *Journal of Traumatic Stress*, *25*, 241–251.

Resnick, S. G., Rosenheck, R. A., & Lehman, A. F. (2004). An exploratory analysis of correlates of recovery. *Psychiatric Services*, *55*, 540–547.

Reupert, A., Maybery, D., Nicholson, J., Gopfert, M., & Seeman, M. V. (Eds.). (2015). *Parental psychiatric disorder: Distressed parents and their families*. Cambridge, UK: Cambridge University Press.

Rivera-Torres, P., Araque-Padilla, R., & Montero-Simó, M. (2013). Job stress across gender: The importance of emotional and intellectual demands and social support in women. *International Journal of Environmental Research and Public Health*, *10*(1), 375–389.

Roberts, T. A., & Gettman, J. Y. (2004). Mere exposure: Gender differences in the negative effects of priming a state of self-objectification. *Sex Roles*, *51*, 17–27.

Robins, C. S., Sauvageot, J. A., Cusack, K. J., Suffoletta-Maierle, S., & Frueh, B. C. (2005). Consumers perceptions of negative experiences and "sanctuary harm" in psychiatric setting. *Psychiatric Services*, *6*, 1134–1138.

Rogers, A. (2015). Strait jackets are still in use, just not where you think. Retrieved from https://science.howstuffworks.com/science-vs-myth/straitjackets-are-still-use-just-not-where-you-think.htm

Rogers, E. S., Anthony, W. A., Toole, J., & Brown, M. A. (1991). Vocational outcomes following psychosocial rehabilitation. *Journal of Vocational Rehabilitation*, *1*(3), 21–29.

Rogers, E. S., Chamberlin, J., Ellison, M. L., & Crean, T. (1997). A consumer-constructed scale to measure empowerment among users of mental health services. *Psychiatric Services, 48*(8), 1042–1047.

Rose, D. (1993). Sexual assault, domestic violence and incest. In D. Stewart & N. Stotland (Eds.), *Psychological aspects of women's health care* (pp. 447–483). Washington, DC: American Psychiatric Press.

Rosenbaum, B., Alberdi, F., Haahr, U., Lindhardt, A., & Urfer-Parnas, A. (2019). [Psychodynamic psychotherapy of patients with schizophrenia spectrum psychosis.] *Ugeskrift for Laeger, 181*(3), V06180425.

Rosenfield, S. (1989). The effects of women's employment: Personal control and sex differences in mental health. *Journal of Health and Social Behavior, 30*, 77–91.

Rowe, M. (2015). *Citizenship and mental health.* New York, NY: Oxford University Press.

Rudman, L. A., & Mescher, K. (2012). Of animals and objects: Men's implicit dehumanization of women and likelihood of sexual aggression. *Personality and Social Psychology Bulletin, 38*(6), 734–746.

Quinn, D. M., Kallen, R. W., & Cathey, C. (2006). Body on my mind: The lingering effect of state self-objectification. *Sex Roles, 55*, 869–874.

Sam, D. L., & Morreira, V. (2012). Revisiting the mutual embeddedness of culture and mental illness. *Online Readings in Psychology and Culture*, Unit 10.2. Retrieved from http://works.bepress.com/david_sam/27

Sanchez, D. T., & Kiefer, A. K. (2007). Body concerns in and out of the bedroom: Implications for sexual pleasure and problems. *Archives of Sexual Behavior, 36*, 808–820.

Sánchez, J., Muller, V., Garcia, M. E., Martinez, S. N., Cool, S. T., & Gandarilla, E. (2017). *Journal of Applied Rehabilitation Counseling, 48*(1), 40–49.

Sands, R. G. (1995). The parenting experience of low-income single women with serious mental disorders. *Families in Society, 76*(2), 86–96.

Saunders, J. (1999). Family functioning in families providing care for a family member with schizophrenia. *Issues in Mental Health Nursing, 20*(2), 95–113.

Scheff, T. (1966). *Being mentally ill: A sociological theory.* Chicago, IL: Aldine.

Seeman, M. V. (2000). Women and schizophrenia. *Medscape Women's Health, 5*(2), 1–8.

Seeman, M. V. (2004). Gender differences in the prescribing of antipsychotic drugs. *American Journal of Psychiatry, 161*, 1324–1333.

Sells, D. J., Stayner, D. A., & Davidson, L. (2004). Recovering the self in schizophrenia: An integrative review of qualitative studies. *Psychiatric Quarterly, 75*, 87–97.

Shafer, A., & Ang, R. (2018). The Mental Health Statistics Improvement Program (MHSIP) Adult Consumer Satisfaction Survey factor structure and relation to external criteria. *Journal of Behavioral Health Services and Research, 9*, 1–14.

Shehata, H. A., & Nelson-Piercy, C. (2001). Drugs in pregnancy: Drugs to avoid. *Best Practices & Research in Clinical Obstetrics & Gynaecology, 15*, 971–986.

Showalter, E. (1995). *The female malady: Women, madness, and English culture, 1830–1980.* London, UK: Virago Press.

Silver, S. (1986). An inpatient program for post-traumatic stress disorder: Context as treatment. In C. Figley (Ed.), *Trauma and its wake, Volume II: Post-traumatic stress disorder: Theory, research and treatment.* New York, NY: Brunner/Mazel.

Skodol, A. E., & Bender, D. S. (2003). Why are women diagnosed borderline more than men? *Psychiatric Quarterly, 74*(4), 349–360.

Slade, M. (2009). *Personal recovery and mental illness: A guide for mental health professionals*. Cambridge, UK: Cambridge University Press.

Smith-Rosenberg, C. (1972). The hysterical woman: Sex roles and role conflict in 19th-century *American Social Research, 39*(4), 652–678.

Smith-Rosenberg, C., & Rosenberg, C. (1973). The female animal: Medical and biological views of woman and her role in nineteenth-century America. *Journal of American History, 60*, 332–356.

Sneddon, A. (2016). Medicine, belief, witchcraft and demonic possession in late seventeenth-century Ulster. *Journal of Medical Humanities, 42*, 81–86.

Snell-Rodd, C., Hauensteing, E., Leukefeld, C., Feltner, F., Marcum, A., & Schoenberg, N. (2017). Mental health treatment seeking patterns and preferences of Appalachian women with depression. *American Journal of Orthopsychiatry, 87*, 233.

Spaniol, L., Wewiorski, N., Gagne, C., & Anthony, W. (2002). The process of recovery from schizophrenia. *International Review of Psychiatry, 14*(4), 327–336.

Spece, R. G. (1972). Conditioning and other technologies used to treat rehabilitate demolish prisoners and mental patients. *Southern California Law Review Library, 45*, 616.

Spielvogel, A. M., & Floyd, A. K. (1997). Assessment of trauma in women psychiatric patients. In M. Harris & C. Landis (Eds.), *Sexual abuse in the lives of women diagnosed with serious mental illness* (pp. 39–64). New York, NY: Brunner-Routledge.

Stansfeld, S., & Candy, B. (2006). Psychosocial work environment and mental health—a meta-analytic review. *Scandinavian Journal of Work, Environment & Health, 32*(6), 443–462.

Steadman, H. J., Osher, F. C., Robbins, P. C., Case, B., & Samuels, S. (2009). Prevalence of serious mental illness among jail inmates. *Psychiatric Services, 60*(6), 761–765.

Steel, C., Hardy, A., Smith, B., Wykes, T., Rose, S., Enright, S., . . . Rose, D. (2017). Cognitive–behaviour therapy for post-traumatic stress in schizophrenia: A randomized controlled trial. *Psychological Medicine, 47*(1), 43–51.

Stein, J. A., Leslie, M. B., & Nyamathi, A. (2002). Relative contributions of parent substance use and childhood maltreatment to chronic homelessness, depression, and substance abuse problems among homeless women: Mediating roles of self-esteem and abuse in adulthood. *Child Abuse & Neglect, 26*, 1011–1027.

Stephan, S. (1995). The protection racket—Violence against women: Psychiatric labeling and the law. In *Dare to vision: Shaping the national agenda for women, abuse and mental health services:* Proceedings of a conference held July 14–16, 1994, in Arlington, VA (pp. 25–30).

Stricker, G., & Gold, J. R. (Eds.). (2013). *Comprehensive handbook of psychotherapy integration*. Springer Science & Business Media.

Substance Abuse and Mental Health Services Administration. (2012). National Registry of Evidence Based Practices. Retrieved from http://nrepp.samhsa.gov/ViewIntervention.aspx?id=258

Substance Abuse and Mental Health Services Administration. (2015). Recovery and recovery support. Retrieved from http://www.samhsa.gov

Sullivan, G. (1993). Sexual dysfunction associated with anti-psychotic medications. *Current Approaches to Psychoses, 5*, 8–9.

Szymanski, D. M., Carr, E. R., & Moffit, L. B. (2011). Sexual objectification of women: Clinical implications and training considerations. *Counseling Psychologist, 39*, 107–126.

Taylor, V., Whittier, N., & Rupp, L. J. (2009). *Feminist frontiers* (8th ed.). New York, NY: McGraw-Hill.

Terry, J. (1999). *An American obsession: Science, medicine, and homosexuality in modern society*. Chicago, IL: University of Chicago Press.

Tew, J., Ramon, S., Slade, M., Bird, V., Melton, J., & Le Boutillier, C. (2012). Social factors and recovery from mental health difficulties: A review of the evidence. *British Journal of Social Work, 42*(3), 443–460.

Tewari, N., & Alvarez, A. N. (2009). *Asian American psychology: Current perspectives*. New York, NY: Taylor & Francis Group.

Thomas, K., & Snowden, L. R. (2001). Minority response to health insurance coverage for mental health problems. *Journal of Mental Health Policy and Economics, 4*, 35–41.

Thomas, N., Komiti, A., & Judd, F. (2014). Pilot early intervention antenatal group program for pregnant women with depression and anxiety. *Archive of Women's Mental Health, 17*, 503–509.

Thompson, A., Singh, S., & Birchwood, M. (2016). Views of early psychosis clinicians on discontinuation of antipsychotic medication following symptom remission in first-episode psychosis. *Early Intervention in Psychiatry, 10*, 355–361.

Thraillkill, J. F. (2002). Doctoring "The Yellow Wallpaper." *English Literary History, 69*(2), 525–566.

Tiggemann, M., & Kuring, J. K. (2004). The role of objectification in disordered eating and depressed mood. *British Journal of Clinical Psychology, 43*, 299–312.

Tomes, N. (1990). Historical perspectives on women and mental illness. In R. D. Apple (Ed.), *Women, health, and medicine in America: A historical handbook*. New York, NY: Garland Publishing, Inc.

Tondora, J., Miller, R., Slade, M., & Davidson, L. (2014). *Partnering for recovery in mental health: A practical guide to person-centered planning*. New York, NY: Wiley Blackwell.

Topor, A., Borg, M., Mezzina, R., Sells, D., Marin, I., & Davidson, L. (2006). Others: The role of family, friends and professionals in the recovery process. *American Journal of Psychiatric Rehabilitation, 9*(1), 17–37.

Torgalsboen, A. K. (1999). Full recovery from schizophrenia: The prognostic role of premorbid adjustment, symptoms at first admission, precipitating events and gender. *Psychiatry Research, 88*, 143–152.

Torrey, E. F., & Yolken, R. H. (2010). Psychiatric genocide: Nazi attempts to eradicate schizophrenia. *Schizophrenia Bulletin, 36*(1), 26–32.

U.S. Department of Health and Human Services. (2003). *Achieving the promise: Transforming mental health care in America. President's New Freedom Commission on Mental Health. Final Report*. Rockville, MD: Substance Abuse and Mental Health Services Administration, U.S. Department of Health and Human Services.

U.S. Department of Health and Human Services. (2005). *Federal action agenda: Transforming mental health care in America*. Rockville, MD: Substance Abuse and Mental Health Services Administration.

Ussher, J. (1991). *Women's madness: Misogyny or mental illness?* Amherst, MA: University of Massachusetts Press.

van der Kolk, B. A. (1987). The psychological consequences of overwhelming life experiences. In B. A. Van der Kolk (Ed.), *Psychological trauma*. Washington, DC: American Psychiatric Press.

van der Kolk, B. A. (1989). The compulsion to repeat the trauma: Re-enactment, revictimization, and masochism. *Psychiatric Clinics of North America, 12*(2), 389–411.

van der Kolk, B. A. (1994). The body keeps score: Memory and the evolving psychobiology of posttraumatic stress. *Harvard Review of Psychiatry,* January/February, 253–265.

Wahl, A. K., Rustoen, T., Lerdal, A., Hanestad, B. R., Knudsen, O., & Moum, T. (2004). The Norwegian version of the Herth Hope Index (HHI-N): A psychometric study. *Palliative and Supportive Care, 2,* 255–263.

Walker, L. (1994). *Abused women and survivor therapy: A practical guide for the psychotherapist.* Washington, DC: American Psychological Association.

Walsh, C., MacMillan, H., & Jamieson, E. (2002). The relationship between parental psychiatric disorder and child physical and sexual abuse: Findings from the Ontario Health Supplement. *Child Abuse & Neglect, 26,* 11–22.

Ware, N., Hopper, K., Tugenberg, T., Dickey, B., & Fisher, D. (2008). A theory of social integration as quality of life. *Psychiatric Services, 59,* 27–33.

Ware, N. C., & Goldfinger, S. M. (1997). Poverty and rehabilitation in severe psychiatric disorders. *Psychiatric Rehabilitation Journal, 21*(1), 3–9.

Wieck, A., & Haddad, P. M. (2003). Antipsychotic-induced hyperprolactinaemia in women: Pathophysiology, severity and consequences: Selective literature review. *British Journal of Psychiatry, 182,* 199–204.

Wilks, S. E., Heintz, M. E., Lemieux, C. M., & Du, X. (2020). Assessing social connectedness among persons with schizophrenia: Psychometric evaluation of the Perceived Social Connectedness Scale. *Journal of Behavioral Health Services & Research, 47*(1), 113–125.

Wilton, R. (2004). Putting policy into practice? Poverty and people with serious mental illness. *Social Science & Medicine, 58,* 25–39.

Winans, E. A. (2001). Antipsychotics and breastfeeding. *Journal of Human Lactation, 17,* 344–347.

Wisconsin Coalition for Advocacy. (1994). *Report on patient treatment concerns and use of restraint and seclusion in violation of Sec. 51.61, Wis. Stats., at the Step Unit, Winnebago Mental Health Institute* (p. 14).

Wisdom, J. P., Bruce, K., Auzeen Saedi, G., Weis, T., & Green, C. A. (2008). "Stealing me from myself": Identity and recovery in personal accounts of mental illness. *Australian & New Zealand Journal of Psychiatry, 42*(6), 489–495.

Wise, T. (2005). *White like me: Reflections on race from a privileged son* (rev. ed.). Berkeley, CA: Soft Skull Press.

Wolff, N., Frueh, B. C., Shi, J., & Schumann, B. E. (2012). Effectiveness of cognitive-behavioral trauma treatment for incarcerated women with mental illnesses and substance abuse disorders. *Journal of Anxiety Disorders, 26,* 703–710.

Wong, Y. L. I., Matejkowski, J., & Lee, S. (2011). Social integration of people with serious mental illness: Network transactions and satisfaction. *Journal of Behavioral Health Services & Research, 38*(1), 51–67.

Woods, N. F. (1985). Employment, family roles, and mental ill health in young married women. *Nursing Research, 34*(1), 1–10.

World Health Organization. (1973). *The international pilot study of schizophrenia.* Geneva, Switzerland: World Health Organization.

Worrell, J., & Remer, P. (2003). *Feminist perspectives in therapy: Empowering diverse women*. Hoboken, NJ: John Wiley & Sons.

Wright, E. R., Wright, D. E., Perry, B. L., & Foote-Ardah, C. E. (2007). Stigma and the sexual isolation of people with serious mental illness. *Social Problems, 54*(1), 78–98.

Wynaden, D., Ladzinski, U., Lapsley, J., Landsborough, I., Butt, J., & Hewitt, V. (2006). The caregiving experience: How much do health professionals understand? *Collegian, 13*(3), 6–10.

Wyska, E., & Jusko, W. J. (2001). Approaches to pharmacokinetic/pharmacodynamic modeling during pregnancy. *Seminars in Perinatology, 25*, 124–132.

Yanos, P. T., Rosenfield, S., & Horwitz, A. V. (2001). Negative and supportive social interactions and quality of life among persons diagnosed with severe mental illness. *Community Mental Health Journal, 37*(5), 405–419.

Ziguras, S., Klimidis, S., Lewis, J., & Stuart, G. (2003). Ethnic matching of clients and clinicians and use of mental health services by ethnic minority clients. *Psychiatric Services, 54*, 535–541.

For the benefit of digital users, indexed terms that span two pages (e.g., 52–53) may, on occasion, appear on only one of those pages.

Tables and figures are indicated by *t* and *f* following the page number

abuse. *See also* retraumatization; sexual abuse; trauma
 denial of, 136
 forgiveness of perpetrators, 144
 intimate partner violence, 53, 59–60, 116
 physical, 116, 117, 132–34
 safety planning, 59–60
Abused Women and Survivor Therapy: A Practical Guide for the Psychotherapist (Walker), 136–38
acceptance and commitment therapy group, 63
acknowledgement of illness, role in recovery, 30
adipose tissue, drug metabolism and, 32
African Americans
 explanatory models of SMI, 94
 mental health disparities, 92–94
 spirituality and religion among, 99–100, 101
agency, role in recovery, 29–30
Aitken, D., 74, 74*t*
alcohol abuse, 72–73, 118–19
Alverson, H. S., 95
American Indians, 92–93, 100
anorexia, 17–18
Anthony, W., 133
antipsychiatry movement, 21
antipsychotic medications, 19–20, 33–34, 53

Asian Americans, 92–93
assessments
 psychological, creation of, 19
 of relationships, 60–61
 of trauma, 154
asylum psychiatry, 11–12
autonomy, 29–30

barriers to help seeking, 136–38
Beard, G. M., 16
bed therapy, 21
behavioral family therapy, 58, 61–62, 124
behavioral strategies, 74
Belicki, K., 144
Belle, D., 75
biological concerns in recovery, 32–35
biological essentialism, 12
bleedings, as nymphomania treatment, 17
body surveillance, 113–14, 118–19
boundaries with clients with trauma histories, 145
Boyle, E. J., 48–49, 49*t*
Braslow, J. T., 19–21
breastfeeding, 34–35
Breuer, J., 15
Brown, I. B., 13–14
Buddhism, 100
bulimia nervosa, 118

caregiving, 47, 51–52, 71
Carpenter-Song, E., 94–95
Charcot, J.-M., 10, 15
Chen, S. X., 93
Cheng, T. C., 93–94
Chesler, P., 6–7, 12, 21
Cheslerian thesis, 6–7
childbirth
    insanity after, 14
    motherhood, 47–50
    postpartum depression, 34–35
childcare, access to, 65
choice in relationships, 50–51, 58–59
Christianity, 99–100
citizenship, rights of, 29
class
    anorexia and, 17–18
    asylum psychiatry, 11
    case narratives, 78–84
    clinical strategies, 87
    financial problems, 75–77, 84–86
    kleptomania and, 18
    mental health and, 75f, 77–78
    neurasthenia and, 16
    overview, 75
    Work and Class Worksheet, 90
Cleaves, M., 16
clitoridectomy, 10, 12, 13–14, 17
cognitive-behavioral treatments, 123–24
colonial United States, mistreatment
    in, 9–10
commitment, role in recovery, 27
community, developing friendships
    in, 65
community action and advocacy, 38,
    151t, 153–54
comorbid physical conditions, 35
compassion fatigue, 144
complex PTSD (C-PTSD), 134–35
conservatorship, 59
contraception, 47
control, role in recovery, 29–30
Cooper, D., 21
coping mechanisms, 74, 99–100, 137
Corrigan, P., 91–92
countertransference trauma, 144
C-PTSD (complex PTSD), 134–35

culture
    case narratives, 102–7
    clinical applications, 108–9
    clinical strategies, 109–10
    Cultural Strengths and Stigma
        Worksheet, 112
    factors for women with SMI, 107–8
    LGBT individuals, 96–97
    race and ethnicity, 91–95
custody of children, 47–48

Darwinian psychiatry, 12
dating, 52–55
DBT (dialectical behavior therapy), 60,
    62, 123–24
DeCourville, N., 144
Deegan, P. E., 55
DeMartini, L., 53–55, 54t
demonological view of mental illness,
    8, 9–10
denial of abuse, 136
depot injections, 32
depression
    postpartum, 34–35
    poverty and, 76
    during pregnancy, 34
    work and, 71–72
Desmond, M., 75–76
developmental concerns in recovery, 32–35
diagnostic dialectic tension, 3
diagnostic mislabeling of trauma, 134
dialectical behavior therapy (DBT), 60,
    62, 123–24
discrimination. See also racism; stigma
    case narratives, 102–3
    explanatory models, 94–95
    of LGBT individuals, 96–97
    types of, 91–92
Dohrenwend, B. P., 77
domestic violence, 53, 59–60, 116
double burden, 71–72
Draijer, N., 133–34
drug interactions, 32
Duckworth, M. P., 132

Eack, S. M., 94
eating disorders, 17–18, 97, 118

egalitarian therapy relationships, 155–56
electroconvulsive therapy (ECT), 19–20
emotional processing, 123–24
empowerment, 29, 38, 55, 62. *See also*
    Women's Empowerment and
    Recovery-Oriented Care
Empowerment Scale, 154
essentialism, biological, 12
ethnicity
    discrimination based on, 91–92
    explanatory models, 94–95
    mental health disparities, 92–94
eugenics, 12, 20
Europe, history of mistreatment in, 9–10
European Americans, 92–93
Evicted (Desmond), 75–76
eviction, 75–76
exercise, 35

Fallot, R. D., 98–99
family
    motherhood, 47–50
    relationships, 51–52
    support from, 26
    work and, 71–72
family consultation, 64
family psychoeducation, 64
family therapy, 63–64
Family-to-Family groups, 63
Female Malady: Women, Madness, and
    English Culture, 1830–1980, The
    (Showalter), 7–8
feminist therapy, 152–53
Finnerty, M., 47–48
first-episode psychosis, 55–56
Follette, V. M., 132
forgiveness of perpetrators of abuse, 144
foundational constructs, 58–60
Freud, S., 14–16, 19
friendship, 50–51, 65
full citizenship, role in recovery, 29

Gabbidon, J., 92
Galen, 9
gender bias in treatment, 3–4, 8
Gender Dysphoria, diagnosis of, 97
gendered workplaces, 73

gender oppression, 3, 15–16
gender roles
    analyses of, 123, 127, 130
    industrialization, effect on, 11
    Masculine-Feminine Test, 19
    in neurasthenia diagnosis, 16
    work and, 73–74, 74*t*
gender-sensitive therapy, 3, 152–53
Gilman, C. P., 16
Goodell, W., 12–13
Goossens, P. J., 133–34
Green, A., 100
group strategies, for relationship
    support, 63–64
Gupta, B. S., 98
Gupta, U., 98
gynecological surgery, 10, 12–14, 17

handicrafts, 11
Hanna, F. J., 100
health insurance, 92–93
healthy worker effect, 72
Heath, C. D., 101
help seeking, barriers to, 136–38
Herman, J., 134, 143, 145
Hildegard of Binge, 9
Hinduism, 100
Hippocrates, 8–9
Hirshbein, L., 12
history of mistreatment. *See* mistreatment,
    history of
holistic care, 40
Holocaust, 20
homelessness, 3, 75–76, 77, 79
homemaker role, 71
hope, role in recovery, 27
hormones, 33–34, 40
Horney, K., 19
hospitalization. *See also* retraumatization
    of African Americans, 94
    asylum psychiatry, 11–12
    psychiatric, 19–20
    sanctuary trauma, 132–33, 135–36
housing problems, 3, 75–76, 77, 79
humorism model, 8–9
hyperprolactinemia, 33
hypnotism, 15

hysterectomy, 17
hysteria, 8–9, 14–16

Ida, D. J., 92–93
identity
  positive sense of, 40
  redefinition of self, 27–28
  relationship challenges, 62–63
immigrant paradox, 93
industrialization, history of mistreatment
      and, 11–18
  anorexia, 17–18
  asylum psychiatry, 11–12
  gynecological surgery, 12–14
  hysteria, 14–16
  kleptomania, 18
  neurasthenia, 16
  nymphomania, 17
  puerperal and lactational insanity, 14
internalized stigma, 96
interpersonal process therapy, 62
interpersonal relationships. See
      relationships
intersectional stigma, 92
  among LGBT individuals, 96–97
  case narratives, 102–7
  work discrimination related to,
      84–85, 85t
intimate partner relationships
  assessment, 60–61
  dating, 52–55
  identity issues, 62–63
  other goals prioritized over, 46
  therapeutic strategies for, 61–62
intimate partner violence, 53, 59–60, 116
Islam, 100

Jennings, A., 132, 135–36
job control, effect on mental health, 72

King, M. L., Jr., 29
Kinsey, A., 17
kleptomania, 18
Kompaniez-Dunigan, E., 48–49, 49t

labiotomies, 12, 13–14, 17
lactational insanity, 12, 14

Laing, R. D., 21
LaMar, K., 53–55, 54t, 74, 74t
Latino Americans
  explanatory models of SMI, 94–95
  mental health disparities, 92–93
  spirituality and religion among, 100
laundry therapy, 11
Lefley, H. P., 64
Lennon, M. C., 72
LGBT individuals
  case narratives, 102–7
  intersectional stigma, 96–97
  Masculine-Feminine Test and, 19
  retraumatization, 138–42
  spirituality and religion among, 100–1
  work and class factors, 78–83
life expectancy, 35
life goals, 28, 30
Lo, C. C., 93–94
lobotomy, 19–20
Logie, C. H., 91
Loughnan, S., 114

madness, theories on history of, 6–8
Mak, W. S., 93
maladaptive coping strategies, 76, 96, 97
Malcolm, W., 144
management of symptoms, 28
marginalization, 25, 26, 29
Masculine-Feminine Test, 19
masturbation, 12–14
matriarchal religions, 101
Mauritz, M. W., 133–34
meaningful activities, role in recovery, 27
medications
  dosage considerations, 32–33
  gender considerations, 32–33
  hormonal changes and, 33
  pregnancy and breastfeeding
      considerations, 34–35
  sexual functioning, effect on, 53
men
  asylum psychiatry, 11
  history of mistreatment of, 8
  hypersexuality in, 17
  hysteria in, 16
  intervention, 156

psychiatric hospitalization of, 19–20
psychotropic medications, response to, 32–33
sexual objectification and, 114–15
sterilization of, 20–21
work and gender, 73
Men's Empowerment and Recovery-Oriented Care (ME-ROC), 156
Merg, A. L., 48–49, 49t
Mesmer, F. A., 15
Miles, C. C., 19
Miller, L., 47–48
minority stress model, 96
misogyny, 105–6
mistreatment, history of
   antipsychiatry movement, 21
   early views on women's mental health, 8–9
   in Europe and colonial United States, 9–10
   industrialization and Victorian era, 11–18
      anorexia, 17–18
      asylum psychiatry, 11–12
      gynecological surgery, 12–14
      hysteria, 14–16
      kleptomania, 18
      neurasthenia, 16
      nymphomania, 17
      puerperal and lactational insanity, 14
   overview, 3–4
   psychiatric hospitalization, 19–20
   sterilization, 20–21
   theoretical perspectives, 6–8
   in 20th century, 18–21
Mizock, L., 48–49, 49t, 53–55, 54t, 74, 74t, 151t, 153–55
M'Mordie, W. K., 12–13
money scripts, 88
Morrow, M., 131
motherhood, 47–50
   breastfeeding, 34–35
   childcare, access to, 65
   custody of children, 47–48
   identity and, 63
   parenting resources, 65
   postpartum depression, 34–35

poverty and eviction, 75–76
Mueser, K. T., 133
multicultural feminist therapy, 62
mutuality in relationships, 51, 52

narrative therapy, 63
National Alliance on Mental Illness (NAMI), 63
Native Americans, 92–93, 100
Nazi sterilization, 20–21
neurasthenia, 16
Newhill, C. E., 94
non-citizenship, 29
nymphomania, 17

objectification theory, 113
ovariectomy, 12–13, 17

Packard, E., 12
parenting resources, 65
Participant Feedback Inventory, 154, 159
peer specialists, 156
penis envy, 19
Perceived Social Connectedness scale, 61
Perese, E., 77–78
person-centered treatment planning, 38–39, 61
physical abuse, 116, 117, 132–34
physical well-being, 35
Pina, A., 114
positive sense of identity, 40
postpartum depression, 34–35
post-traumatic stress disorder (PTSD)
   case narratives, 118–20
   clinical treatments, 123–24
   complex PTSD, 134–35
   diagnosis of, 117
   prevalence rates of, 116
   retraumatization case narratives, 139
   Seeking Safety intervention for, 150
poverty
   harmful effects of, 75
   mental health and, 77–78
   women and, 75–77
pregnancy, 34–35, 47–50
Primm, A. B., 92–93
privacy in psychiatric units, 31

prolactin levels, 32–33
provider revictimization, 137
psychiatric hospitalization, 19–20,
        31, 132–33
psychiatric modernism, 21
psychiatrists, sexual abuse by, 21
psychoeducational support
        groups, 64
psychological assessments, 19
psychological incest, 21
psychological trauma, 115
psychotherapy integration, 62
psychotropic medications, 32–33
PTSD. *See* post-traumatic stress disorder
puerperal insanity, 12, 14
Puvia, E., 114

race
    discrimination, 91–92
    explanatory models of SMI, 94–95
    mental health disparities, 92–94
racism, 91–92, 94–95
    case narratives, 102–3
rape, 114, 118–20
RAS (Recovery Assessment Scale), 154
reciprocity in relationships, 51, 52
recovery, 2–3. *See also* Women's
        Empowerment and
        Recovery-Oriented Care
    acknowledgement of illness, 30
    biological and developmental
        concerns, 32–35
    case narratives, 35–38
    citizenship rights and, 29
    clinical applications, 38–40
    clinical strategies, 41
    control and agency, 29–30
    defining, 25–26
    hope and commitment in, 27
    hormonal factors, 33–34
    life expectancy, 35
    meaningful activities and valued social
        roles in, 27
    medications in, 32–33
    My Recovery Journey Worksheet, 44
    overview, 24
    physical well-being, 35

pregnancy and breastfeeding
        considerations, 34–35
    programming, 31
    redefinition of self, 27–28
    from sanctuary trauma, 133
    spirituality and religion in, 98
    support from others, 26
    symptom management, 28
Recovery Assessment Scale (RAS), 154
redefinition of self, role in recovery, 27–28
relationships
    assessment of, 60–61
    case narratives, 55–58
    choice in, 58–59
    clinical strategies, 66–67
    complexities in, 55
    dating, 52–55
    family, 51–52
    foundational constructs, 58–60
    friendship, 50–51
    general discussion, 45–47
    group strategies for, 63–64
    identity issues, 62–63
    motherhood, 47–50
    Relationship Structuring Worksheet, 69
    resources for, 64–65
    safety in, 59–60
    support for, 60
    therapeutic strategies, 61–62
    treatment planning, 61
religion
    benefits on mental health, 97–99
    case narratives, 103–4, 106–7
    clinical applications, 108–9
    clinical strategies, 109–10
    cultural differences in, 99–101
    religious delusions, 99
    transcendental experiences, 99
    women and, 101, 107–8
reproductive system
    gynecological surgery, 10, 12–14, 17
    hormonal changes, 33–34
    hysteria associated with, 8–9
    puerperal and lactational insanity, 14
    sex hormones, mental illness associated
        with, 18
    sterilization, 20–21

resilience, 24, 73, 95, 99–101
rest cure, 16
retraumatization
    barriers to help seeking, 136–38
    case narratives, 138–42
    clinical applications, 142–45
    clinical strategies, 145–46
    conceptualization of, 132–33
    in mental health services, 135–36
    overview, 131–32
    preventing, 124, 142–45, 148
    trauma assessment, 134–35
    women and, 133–34
*Retraumatization: Assessment, Treatment,
    and Prevention* (Duckwork and
    Follette), 132
revictimization, provider, 137
rights of citizenship, role in recovery, 29
romantic relationships
    assessment of, 60–61
    dating, 52–55
    identity issues, 62–63
    intimate partner violence, 53,
        59–60, 116
    other goals prioritized over, 46
    therapeutic strategies for, 61–62
Rosen, J., 21
Rosenfield, S., 72
Ruggiero, Trotula de, 9

safety in relationships, 59–60
Salem witch trials in New England, 10
SAMSHA (Substance Abuse and
    Mental Health Services
    Administration), 25–26
sanctuary trauma, 132–33, 135–36. *See
    also* retraumatization
satyriasis, 17
schizophrenia, 32, 35, 45–46, 53, 117
second shift, 71–72
Seeking Safety intervention, 150
segregation of genders in health care, 17
self, redefinition of, 27–28
self-blame, 136
self-care, 144
self-direction, 30
self-objectification, 113–15

self-stigma, 96
SES. *See* socioeconomic status
sex hormones, mental illness associated
    with, 18
sexism, 102–3, 105–6
sexual abuse
    case narratives, 118–20
    gender disparity in, 117, 133–34
    by psychiatrists, 21
    retraumatization, 131, 138–42
    sanctuary trauma, 132–33
    sexual objectification and, 114
sexual behavior
    dating, 52–55
    gynecological surgery to
        correct, 20–21
    hysteria associated with, 8–9
    nymphomania, 17
    safe sex and contraceptive use, 47
sexual objectification
    case narratives, 118–22
    clinical applications, 122–25
    clinical strategies, 126–28
    general discussion, 113–15
    impact on women, 117–18
    trauma and, 117–18
shared decision-making models, 38–39
shift work, 72–73
Showalter, E., 7–8, 12, 21
Silver, S., 132–33
smelling salts, 15
social capital, 85
social causation models, 77
social-economic stress model, 77
social justice, 41, 101, 117, 125, 127
social network. *See* social support
social resources, 64–65
social roles, 27, 65, 114
social selection models, 77
social skills training group, 63
social status, 76
social support
    friendships, 50–51
    for LGBT individuals, 96
    resources, 64–65
    in workplace, 72–73
social withdrawal, 77–78

socioeconomic status (SES)
    mental health and, 77–78
    women and, 75–77
Soranus, 9
spiritual explanatory models of mental
        illness, 8, 9–10
spirituality
    among women, 101, 107–8
    benefits on mental health, 97–99
    case narratives, 103–4, 106–7
    clinical applications, 108–9
    clinical strategies, 109–10
    cultural differences in, 99–101
    Cultural Strengths and Stigma
            Worksheet, 112
    religious delusions, 99
    spiritual genogram, 111f
Starks, S. L., 19–20
sterilization, 12–13, 20–21
stigma
    among LGBT individuals, 96–97
    explanatory models of SMI, 94–95
    intersectional, 84–85
    poverty and, 77
    social isolation, 26, 29
Stringer, J., 53–55, 54t
substance abuse, 97, 118–19, 150
Substance Abuse and Mental Health
        Services Administration
        (SAMSHA), 25–26
suicidality
    among transgender individuals, 97
    eviction and, 75–76
    interpersonal dynamics and, 56–58
    retraumatization case narratives, 139
    trauma and, 118–20, 123–24
supernatural sorcery, mental illness
        associated with, 8, 9–10
support
    family relationships, 51–52
    friendships, 50–51
    in relationships, 60
    role in recovery, 26
supported employment, gender differences
        in, 73–74
surgeries
    gynecological, 10, 12–14, 17

lobotomy, 19–20
sterilization, 20–21
symptom management, role in recovery, 28

TARGET (Trauma Affect Regulation:
        Guide for Education and
        Therapy), 124
Terman, L., 19
Thomas Aquinas, St., 9
Tomes, N., 7, 13
Tondora, J., 25
transcendental experiences, 99
transgender individuals, 97. See also LGBT
        individuals
transportation services, 65
transtheoretical stages of change model, 60
trauma. See also post-traumatic stress
        disorder; retraumatization
    assessment of, 134–35
    case narratives, 118–22
    clinical applications, 122–25
    defined, 115
    gender and, 117–18
    prevalence rates of, 116
    SMI and, 116–17
    vicarious, 144
Trauma Affect Regulation: Guide
        for Education and Therapy
        (TARGET), 124
Trauma and Recovery (Herman), 134
trauma assessment, 134–35
20th century, history of mistreatment
        in, 18–21

understanding of illness, role in
        recovery, 30
unmet needs, 77–78
Ussher, J., 6–7, 8, 10, 17–18

valued social roles, 27, 65
Values in Action Inventory of Strengths
        (VIAS), 61
van Achterberg, T., 133–34
vasectomies, 20–21
Vasquez, E. A., 114
vicarious trauma, 144
victim blaming, 134, 136

Victorian era, mistreatment during, 11–18
  anorexia, 17–18
  asylum psychiatry, 11–12
  gynecological surgery, 12–14
  hysteria, 14–16
  kleptomania, 18
  neurasthenia, 16
  nymphomania, 17
  puerperal and lactational insanity, 14
violence toward women, 77. *See also* sexual
      abuse; trauma
  intimate partner violence, 53,
      59–60, 116
  physical abuse, 116, 117, 132–34

Walker, L., 136–38, 143
weight gain, due to medications, 33
Wellness Recovery Action Plan (WRAP)
      group, 39
WE-ROC. *See* Women's Empowerment
      and Recovery-Oriented Care
Weyer, J., 10
White Americans, 95, 104
White privilege, 76, 104
witchcraft, mental illness associated
      with, 9–10
witness guilt, 144
womanist spiritual tradition, 101
women-centered religions, 101

Women's Empowerment and Recovery-
      Oriented Care (WE-ROC), 5, 145
  clinical applications, 155–56
  clinical strategies list, 156–57
  intervention framework, 150–53
  Participant Feedback Inventory, 159
  pilot study, 153–55
  recovery assessment measures, 154
  treatment modules, 151*t*, 153
  treatment research, 149–50
*Women's Madness: Misogyny or Mental
      Illness?* (Ussher), 6–7, 8
work
  benefits on mental health, 70–71
  case narratives, 78–84
  clinical strategies, 87
  control in workplace, 72
  family roles, 71–72
  gendered workplaces, 73
  overview, 70–71
  social support, 72–73
  women with SMI and, 73–74, 74*t*, 84–86
  Work and Class Worksheet, 90
worker protections, 85
World Health Organization, 24
WRAP (Wellness Recovery Action Plan)
      group, 39

Yellow Wallpaper, The (Gilman), 16